AF407037

Uncharted Midlife

On the Crossroads of
Aging and Disability

Dr Abha Khetarpal

About the book

This book focuses on the never discussed topic of midlife crisis of persons with disabilities and how the challenges can be managed.

Acknowledgement

I would like to thank to all the individuals with disabilities who shared their personal stories of midlife challenges.

Website: www.abhakhetarpal.com

Email: abha.khetarpal@gmail.com

Year of Publishing: 2024

Place: New Delhi, India

Preface

Midlife can be a challenging, introspective phase, filled with change, questions, and, often, a search for deeper meaning. For years, discussions around midlife crises have largely centred on common societal narratives—the stereotypical images of fast cars, career shifts, or "finding oneself" after years of following a prescribed path. But where is the conversation for those of us who approach midlife while living with a disability? What about our unique challenges, our fears, our dreams, and our questions? How do we navigate the crossroads of aging and disability when the world barely acknowledges our journey?

This book was born out of those questions and the profound need to fill a void. As a woman with a disability experiencing my own midlife crisis, I have found myself in uncharted territory. I know I am not alone; yet, I rarely see reflections of my experiences in books, media, or even in conversations with friends and family. Many of us living with disabilities face an added layer of complexity as we navigate midlife: the physical and emotional challenges of aging are often compounded by the unique realities of our disabilities. We may face changes in mobility, an increased reliance on others for care, the fear of losing independence, or even a sense of isolation and invisibility as the world around us moves on. These issues affect us deeply, shaping how we see ourselves and how we move forward.

I believe managing a midlife crisis is not just a matter of survival but an essential path toward reclaiming quality of life and nurturing our inner resilience. Through honest reflection, shared stories, and practical guidance, I hope this book opens up a long-overdue dialogue around the midlife experiences of people with disabilities. This book is my way of reaching out to others who, like me, are walking this unmarked road. It is my invitation to find strength in shared experiences and to explore the possibilities that midlife holds—even if those possibilities look different from traditional narratives.

In these pages, you will find discussions on the emotional, psychological, and practical challenges that people with disabilities face in midlife. We'll examine the role of mental health, the importance of physical care, and strategies for adapting to the changing needs that come with aging. We'll talk about maintaining independence, finding fulfilment, and nurturing relationships. And, just as importantly, we'll explore how to build a future with dignity, purpose, and self-compassion.

This book is for anyone who feels unseen in their journey through midlife, who is searching for answers, or who simply wants to feel understood. I hope that by bringing these issues to light, we can build a foundation of support, compassion, and empowerment for people with disabilities facing midlife challenges. In the words of the poet Rainer Maria Rilke, "Live the questions now. Perhaps you will then gradually, without noticing it, live along some distant day into the answer."

Together, let's begin that journey.

Dr. Abha Khetarpal

Who is this book for?

This book has a broad potential audience, each of whom could gain valuable insights and guidance.

1. Individuals with Disabilities

Benefit: This group is at the core of the book's purpose. For individuals with disabilities, particularly those in or approaching midlife, this book provides validation, understanding, and practical tools to manage the emotional challenges unique to this stage of life.

Why: It can be empowering for readers to see their experiences represented and to understand that their feelings are shared by others. The book offers insights into managing issues such as shifting identities, career limitations, changes in independence, and fears about aging, making it a valuable personal resource.

2. Family Members and Friends

Benefit: This book helps family members and friends understand the midlife crisis experience for loved ones with disabilities, providing insights into how best to offer support during difficult times.

Why: Friends and family are often first to notice changes or signs of a midlife crisis. By understanding triggers, signs, and coping strategies, they can better empathize with their loved ones and offer meaningful assistance or guidance when needed. The book can help them navigate conversations around complex emotions and strengthen their support role.

3. Healthcare Providers (Doctors, Therapists, Counsellors)

Benefit: Healthcare professionals can use the book to gain a disability-informed perspective on midlife crises, expanding their knowledge and approach to better serve this unique population.

Why: Many healthcare providers may not fully understand the intersection between disability and midlife challenges. This book offers them an in-depth look at how disability affects psychological and emotional health during midlife, enabling them to provide more nuanced, supportive, and compassionate care.

4. Social Workers and Case Managers

Benefit: Social workers and case managers often work closely with individuals with disabilities to connect them with resources and support services. This book can deepen their understanding of midlife crisis symptoms and provide them with tools to guide clients through difficult transitions.

Why: Social workers and case managers can play a pivotal role in helping clients navigate life changes by identifying helpful resources, offering crisis intervention, or providing referrals. With a better understanding of midlife issues specific to disability, they can address their clients' needs more effectively.

5. Employers and Human Resource Professionals

Benefit: This book can serve as an educational resource for HR professionals, managers, and employers, helping them foster a more supportive, inclusive work environment for employees with disabilities.

Why: Midlife crises often intersect with career issues, such as shifts in ambition, ability, or job satisfaction. By understanding these potential struggles, employers and HR professionals can create policies, accommodations, and mental health support systems that address the unique needs of employees with disabilities.

6. Disability Advocates and Nonprofit Organizations

Benefit: Disability advocates and nonprofit organizations can use the book to better understand the challenges faced by people with disabilities in midlife, which can inform advocacy efforts, program development, and public awareness campaigns.

Why: By highlighting this often-ignored issue, advocates and nonprofits can work towards more comprehensive services, including mental health resources, support groups, and educational programs, tailored to the midlife phase for people with disabilities. This knowledge can also support campaigns for policy changes and funding for resources that address these specific needs.

7. Academic Researchers and Students

Benefit: Researchers and students in fields such as psychology, disability studies, social work, and public health can use this book as a foundational text for studying midlife crises in the context of disability.

Why: The book could address an under-researched area, making it a valuable resource for understanding the complex interplay between disability and aging. It could inspire further research, publications, and academic discussion around the emotional and social needs of individuals with disabilities in midlife.

8. Policy Makers and Public Health Officials

Benefit: Policy makers and public health officials can benefit from the book's insights when designing inclusive policies, community resources, and mental health services that address the unique challenges of aging with a disability.

Why: By understanding the unique midlife issues people with disabilities face, these professionals can create more effective, targeted policies and allocate funding to develop programs that support this population. This book could serve as a reference in developing disability-inclusive policies and initiatives for mental health and aging.

Chapter 1: What is a Midlife Crisis, and Why Does It Matter?

Understanding the Midlife Crisis for Persons with Disabilities: A Transformative Phase

The term "midlife crisis" often conjures images of sudden, drastic changes—a middle-aged person leaving a stable career, buying a sports car, or dramatically altering their lifestyle. But for persons with disabilities, the midlife crisis often carries additional layers of complexity, shaped by factors unique to their lived experience. Originally coined by psychologist Elliott Jaques in 1965, the concept of a midlife crisis refers to a period of emotional and psychological turmoil that typically arises between the ages of 40 and 60. This phase often prompts individuals to reflect on their past choices, future aspirations, and overall life trajectory with a heightened sense of urgency.

For people with disabilities, however, this midlife reflection can bring additional questions and challenges that intersect with societal attitudes, physical limitations, evolving support needs, and internalized perceptions of identity. Midlife, for many with disabilities, represents a pivotal juncture where one might confront questions not only about what's been achieved but also about the role disability has played in shaping one's experiences, opportunities, and self-image.

This unique dual perspective—looking back at life while navigating an uncertain future—may provoke profound, and often disability-specific, questions:

- o Has my disability defined me too much, or have I embraced my identity authentically?
- o Have societal expectations limited my choices, or have I found ways to transcend them?
- o What does the future hold for my independence, health, and relationships?

These questions may be accompanied by a complex mix of emotions, from regret to determination, from uncertainty to renewed hope. By recognizing how disability-specific factors influence this life stage, individuals with disabilities can transform their midlife crisis from a period of doubt and struggle into one of meaningful self-discovery and empowerment.

Chapter 2: Why the Midlife Crisis of Persons with Disabilities Gets Ignored

The midlife crisis for individuals with disabilities is often dismissed, overshadowed by stereotypes, societal misconceptions, and systemic barriers that prevent a full understanding of their needs. This chapter explores why this issue is so frequently overlooked, especially in countries like India, where societal expectations and support systems may be particularly narrow.

Societal Misconceptions and Stereotypes

People with disabilities are often seen primarily through the lens of their disability, which can obscure their personal complexities and individual experiences. Society tends to assume that their lives are defined either by constant struggle or by a need for physical accommodations alone. Additionally, there's a common belief that people with disabilities are "used to" adversity, leading to their emotional and psychological struggles being trivialized or dismissed. This creates a misleading narrative that limits understanding of the multifaceted lives of people with disabilities, including the emotional challenges they may face in midlife.

Lack of Inclusive Mental Health Support

Mental health frameworks frequently lack inclusivity when it comes to the specific needs of individuals with disabilities. Counseling and therapy often fail to account for the intersection of disability with life-stage challenges, such as a midlife crisis. Therapists trained in disability-informed care are rare, so many professionals may not fully understand the nuanced concerns of people with disabilities, leaving them without tailored support. This leads to feelings of isolation and alienation, as their emotional struggles remain unacknowledged.

Limited Research and Awareness

Research on midlife crises generally centers on neurotypical individuals, with limited focus on how disability shapes the experience. The lack of data results in a minimal understanding of how midlife transitions uniquely impact people with disabilities. Without robust research, society lacks awareness and resources tailored to their needs, perpetuating a cycle of neglect and limited support networks.

Internalized Stigma and Resilience Expectations

People with disabilities are often portrayed as resilient or "inspirational" simply for navigating daily life, which places immense pressure on them to remain stoic. Expressions of dissatisfaction or crisis may be suppressed, as acknowledging these feelings can feel like a failure to live up to societal expectations. This dynamic can lead individuals to downplay their own experiences, causing them to suffer silently rather than seeking support, as they fear judgment or misunderstanding.

Overemphasis on Physical Health Concerns

Medical professionals and support networks often prioritize physical health, overlooking emotional and psychological needs. This focus on physical well-being inadvertently marginalizes the mental health challenges that may arise, particularly during midlife. The assumption that physical accommodations suffice ignores the broader identity shifts and internal conflicts many individuals face, leaving their midlife crises inadequately addressed.

Social and Economic Barriers

Economic challenges are a significant yet often invisible aspect of midlife crises for people with disabilities. Limited employment opportunities, income constraints, and restricted access to social opportunities compound their stress during midlife transitions.

These financial pressures, along with the high costs of adaptive devices or long-term care, contribute to emotional struggles that are often overshadowed by more immediate economic concerns.

Underdeveloped Support Systems for Middle Age

Support systems for people with disabilities tend to focus on early life stages, such as childhood interventions, education, and initial career support, but rarely extend to address midlife challenges. This leaves people with disabilities without guidance as they encounter evolving aspirations and challenges unique to middle age. The lack of ongoing, age-specific support makes it easy for caregivers, professionals, and even families to overlook the unique struggles faced during this life stage.

Interplay Between Disability and Aging

The challenges of aging are compounded for people with disabilities, who often experience age-related changes alongside disability-related complications. As they encounter increased physical limitations, changes in support needs, and the loss of loved ones, their mental health can be deeply affected. Yet, the societal narrative around aging seldom considers how these combined effects might intensify midlife crises for individuals with lifelong disabilities.

In conclusion, the midlife crisis of individuals with disabilities is often unacknowledged due to a combination of systemic biases, insufficient research, and societal misconceptions. Addressing this gap requires comprehensive changes in mental health care, disability-focused research, and a shift toward inclusive approaches to aging. By recognizing and validating the unique midlife experiences of people with disabilities, society can foster more supportive environments and better equip individuals to navigate this often-overlooked life stage.

Chapter 3: Unique Signs and Symptoms for Persons with Disabilities

A midlife crisis is not a universal experience, and it doesn't manifest the same way for everyone. People with disabilities may experience this phase differently, influenced by the intersecting challenges of physical health changes, accessibility, and shifting support networks. Understanding some of the common signs and symptoms, especially those unique to persons with disabilities, can provide valuable insights for navigating this life stage constructively.

For some, symptoms may appear in emotional forms, such as sadness, dissatisfaction, or an intensified sense of "what if?" stemming from real or perceived limitations encountered over a lifetime. Others might experience outward expressions of change, which could include shifts in lifestyle, health routines, or a re-evaluation of relationships and social supports. People with disabilities might also face a heightened awareness of aging and the potential for increased health needs, a factor that can intensify feelings of vulnerability or prompt a re-evaluation of long-term plans.

Being aware of these signals encourages self-awareness and can motivate individuals to seek support, whether through family, community resources, or mental health professionals who understand the unique intersections of disability and midlife challenges. Recognizing the signs is essential to reframing a midlife crisis as a transformative opportunity—a moment of clarity that invites meaningful reflection on one's identity, desires, and long-term vision.

Recognizing the Signs and Symptoms of a Midlife Crisis for Persons with Disabilities

The signs and symptoms of a midlife crisis can vary widely, yet many people experience common emotional, behavioral, and physical changes during this period. For individuals with disabilities, these signs often reflect not only universal life concerns but also unique experiences tied to disability-related challenges, societal perceptions, and the effects of aging on health and independence. By understanding these symptoms through a disability-focused lens, individuals can gain clarity, foster self-awareness, and respond thoughtfully to this transformative life phase.

Emotional Symptoms: Navigating Inner Turmoil with a Disability Lens

One of the hallmarks of a midlife crisis is a shift in emotional well-being, often marked by intense and sometimes contradictory feelings. For individuals with disabilities, emotional symptoms may also intersect with questions about identity, autonomy, and the role of disability in shaping life's trajectory.

Common emotional symptoms include:

Increased Self-Doubt and Questioning: For individuals with disabilities, midlife may intensify questioning around past choices, including decisions influenced by external expectations or perceived limitations. Comparing personal achievements with societal standards may create additional feelings of inadequacy or prompt reflection on how disability has shaped one's path.

Feeling Unfulfilled or "Stuck": Midlife often brings a sense of stagnation, and for people with disabilities, this may be amplified by external factors such as limited career mobility, social isolation, or accessibility barriers. This period may raise questions about purpose, adaptability, and potential for new experiences that align with evolving abilities and interests.

Intense Reflection on Mortality and Legacy: Aging may bring heightened concerns about future health, independence, and the support needed to maintain a fulfilling life. For some, this introspection extends to how they'll be remembered—not only for their accomplishments but also for their resilience, contributions, and impact within their community and family.

Mood Swings and Emotional Instability: As with many people in midlife, individuals with disabilities may experience fluctuating emotions, but these may be exacerbated by the strain of managing disability-related challenges. This emotional volatility often involves processing regret, resilience, and, at times, pride in overcoming adversity.

These emotional symptoms can serve as motivators for deep introspection, encouraging individuals with disabilities to reassess values, address long-standing questions, and connect with sources of personal meaning that resonate in this life stage.

Behavioural Symptoms: Outward Expressions of Change

In addition to emotional shifts, a midlife crisis often involves noticeable changes in behaviour. For people with disabilities, these behaviours may reflect both the desire to embrace change and the practical need to adapt to evolving abilities and resources.

Common behavioural signs include:

Impulsive or Risky Behaviour: Some individuals might respond to feelings of stagnation or frustration with impulsive actions—such as changing careers, relocating, or undertaking ambitious new projects. This behaviour can stem from a desire to regain autonomy or redefine what freedom means in the context of their disability.

Seeking Novelty or Adventure: People with disabilities may seek new hobbies, relationships, or activities that align with their interests and capabilities. This search often includes adaptive sports, accessible travel, or creative pursuits, providing an empowering sense of adventure that balances personal growth with physical considerations.

Changes in Social Patterns: Shifts in social dynamics are common in midlife. Some individuals may become more introverted, focusing on self-reflection, while others might reach out to create new friendships or reconnect with old ones. These changes are often driven by the desire for meaningful connection and understanding, especially with people who relate to the unique experiences of living with a disability.

Altered Spending Habits: For some, financial behaviour may shift as they invest in health, accessibility, or lifestyle changes to improve quality of life. Others might make purchases related to hobbies, equipment, or experiences that offer a sense of novelty and independence, redefining spending patterns in ways that support both personal and physical needs.

These behavioral changes are often attempts to reassert control, explore identity, and find fulfillment within the context of one's abilities and constraints. Recognizing these signs allows individuals with disabilities to make balanced choices that align with their evolving goals and values.

Physical Symptoms: The Body's Response to Midlife and Disability

Midlife introspection often brings physical manifestations, and for individuals with disabilities, these symptoms can be particularly nuanced. Stress, aging, and disability-related health concerns can converge, influencing physical well-being in ways that reflect the emotional weight of this life stage.

Common physical symptoms include:

Health and Appearance Concerns: Heightened awareness of aging may prompt individuals to focus on physical fitness, health routines, or adaptive self-care practices. Many individuals with disabilities use midlife as a time to reconsider health management strategies, balancing the desire for vitality with realistic expectations.

Fatigue and Changes in Sleep Patterns: Emotional stress and introspection can disrupt sleep patterns, leading to fatigue or altered energy levels. Those with disabilities may find that managing both midlife stress and health-related symptoms creates a compounding effect, impacting rest and overall energy.

Physical Tension and Stress-Related Ailments: The combined emotional and physical strain may result in headaches, muscle tension, or other stress-related ailments. Managing disability and health challenges alongside midlife stress can intensify these symptoms, underscoring the importance of self-care practices tailored to individual needs.

Being attuned to these physical signs is essential, as it can prompt individuals to prioritize adaptive self-care and seek support when needed.

Cognitive and Existential Symptoms: A Shift in Mindset with Disability Perspectives

Beyond emotional and physical changes, a midlife crisis often brings cognitive and existential shifts. For individuals with disabilities, these shifts may include re-evaluating beliefs, identity, and purpose in ways that reflect the unique influence of disability on one's life path.

Common cognitive and existential symptoms include:

Deepened Self-Reflection on Identity: Midlife can prompt individuals with disabilities to reconsider aspects of their identity beyond their disability, exploring how resilience, creativity, and adaptability have contributed to their character.

Reassessment of Beliefs and Values: For some, midlife encourages a re-evaluation of core beliefs and values, especially as they relate to independence, interdependence, and societal expectations. This can bring about a profound shift in understanding what matters most and where to focus energy moving forward.

Heightened Need for Meaning and Purpose: Individuals with disabilities may seek new sources of purpose, often turning to creative outlets, advocacy, or volunteerism that align with personal values and life experiences. This period of exploration can provide a renewed sense of fulfilment.

Recognizing these cognitive and existential signs can help individuals understand that their questions are a natural part of growth and self-discovery. This introspective journey offers people with disabilities the chance to redefine their path with clarity, resilience, and purpose.

Cognitive Symptoms: A Mindset in Flux for Persons with Disabilities

The cognitive shifts experienced during a midlife crisis often lead individuals to re-examine past choices and personal milestones. For persons with disabilities, this self-reflection is often informed by unique experiences of overcoming obstacles, navigating accessibility challenges, and balancing independence with support. Cognitive symptoms in this context reveal deeper reflections on resilience, identity, and the broader impacts of living with a disability.

Increased Self-Reflection and Introspection

Midlife often brings a heightened focus on past choices, and for people with disabilities, this introspection may include evaluating how much disability has shaped life decisions, self-concept, and relationships. Reflecting on "what if" scenarios, they may ponder how different circumstances, improved accessibility, or less societal stigma might have affected their journey. This self-reflection, though challenging, can foster growth and provide new insights into ways to advocate for themselves and pursue unfulfilled dreams.

Preoccupation with Mortality and Legacy

Midlife brings an increased awareness of aging and its impact on health and autonomy. For individuals with disabilities, this reflection can include practical concerns about future care, changes in accessibility, and the need for reliable support networks. Questions of legacy also arise, as individuals may consider how their life, achievements, and resilience have contributed to their family and community. This awareness often fuels a desire to create lasting contributions or to mentor others facing similar challenges.

Desire for Purpose and Meaning

For many with disabilities, the drive for purpose and meaning becomes particularly poignant, as they seek to balance personal goals with practical limitations. This phase often involves a reassessment of prior goals and a search for new ones that feel more attainable and deeply fulfilling. Creative pursuits, disability advocacy, and volunteer work become avenues for exploring purpose, allowing individuals to express values that may have taken a backseat to more immediate concerns earlier in life.

Questioning Long-Held Beliefs and Values

Midlife introspection often brings cognitive dissonance as individuals re-evaluate beliefs shaped by society's perceptions of disability. This period may prompt individuals to challenge assumptions about what they "should" be able to achieve or how much support they "should" need. This re-evaluation process offers an opportunity to shed limiting beliefs, fostering a mindset that honors both autonomy and interdependence in ways that feel authentic.

Decision-Making Difficulties

For people with disabilities, decision-making during a midlife crisis may include complex considerations such as accessibility, healthcare, and financial planning. The desire to change life paths or embrace new pursuits can be accompanied by worries about support structures and future health. This cognitive overload can lead to hesitation, but it also presents an opportunity to make empowered choices that consider both current needs and long-term goals.

Existential Symptoms: The Search for Self and Significance with a Disability Perspective

Existential symptoms of a midlife crisis are often magnified for individuals with disabilities, as they grapple with questions around identity, missed opportunities, and the search for authentic self-expression. For many, these reflections are deeply tied to how disability has influenced personal growth, relationships, and societal contributions.

Existential Anxiety

The awareness of aging can amplify existential anxiety, particularly for those with disabilities who may have increased health considerations or support needs. This anxiety often involves contemplating future independence, care arrangements, and the fulfillment of personal dreams. While this awareness can feel overwhelming, it can also motivate individuals to focus on creating meaningful experiences and to seek reassurance through spirituality, philosophy, or connection with others.

Sense of "Lost" Identity

A midlife crisis often brings questions about identity, and for persons with disabilities, this includes reconciling self-image with societal expectations. Many find themselves reflecting on whether they've been fully recognized for who they are beyond their disability. This period of introspection offers an opportunity to define or redefine an authentic identity, which might involve exploring passions set aside due to societal pressures or physical limitations.

Fear of Wasted Time and Missed Opportunities

Midlife often brings a sense of urgency, especially for people who feel their disability limited certain opportunities. This awareness can provoke regret over goals not pursued or dreams left unexplored. However, this reflection can also serve as a powerful motivator to reclaim those dreams or adapt them to the current reality. This sense of urgency can inspire individuals to take steps toward unfulfilled aspirations, whether through advocacy, creative expression, or new personal projects.

Longing for Authenticity and Self-Expression

As they reassess their lives, individuals with disabilities often develop a heightened desire to live authentically, free from societal expectations that may have shaped past decisions. This longing for authenticity can be liberating, encouraging them to embrace activities, lifestyles, or relationships that align with their core values and individual sense of self.

Spiritual or Philosophical Exploration

The midlife period often sparks a search for meaning, leading individuals with disabilities to explore spiritual or philosophical beliefs that provide comfort, connection, or purpose. For many, this exploration includes advocacy for disability rights, deepening relationships, or connecting with spiritual communities. This phase of introspection offers a chance to affirm a sense of belonging within a larger purpose, empowering individuals to face the future with renewed clarity.

Relational and Social Symptoms: Navigating Changing Connections for Persons with Disabilities

The midlife crisis experience often influences social and familial relationships, prompting a re-evaluation of how these connections align with an individual's evolving sense of self. For people with disabilities, this relational introspection may involve balancing desires for independence, the need for support, and the desire for authentic connections.

Shifts in Marital or Partnership Dynamics

For individuals with disabilities, a midlife crisis may prompt questions about intimacy, autonomy, and compatibility within their partnerships. Reassessing these dynamics can reveal a desire for both independence and mutual support. Open communication about needs and goals is essential, as both partners navigate changing perspectives on shared responsibilities and personal growth.

Reassessment of Intimacy and Compatibility: Some individuals may feel a need to redefine relationship roles, fostering a balance of independence and interdependence that respects evolving needs. This period offers an opportunity for honest dialogue, strengthening connection and mutual understanding.

Exploring New Forms of Relationship Satisfaction: Many seek ways to reignite romance or shared activities that are accessible and enjoyable. Counseling or support groups can be valuable for couples, providing tools to reconnect and support each other through life transitions.

Changes in Friendships and Social Networks

As individuals with disabilities move through midlife, friendships may evolve to reflect their current values and lifestyle needs.

Re-evaluation of Friendships: Some long-standing friendships may no longer feel relevant or supportive. This period often involves a shift toward connections with others who share similar experiences or interests, allowing for greater authenticity.

Desire for Authentic Connections: A midlife crisis often intensifies the desire for meaningful social bonds, encouraging individuals to seek out friends with whom they can share their journey. This shift may involve joining disability advocacy groups or other supportive communities that offer understanding and solidarity.

Renewed Focus on Social Contribution and Community Involvement: Midlife often brings a desire to make an impact, and for people with disabilities, this may manifest through involvement in community projects, advocacy, or mentoring. These activities provide fulfillment and foster a sense of purpose beyond personal relationships.

Family Role Reconfiguration

For individuals with disabilities, family dynamics during midlife may shift as they balance personal needs with family expectations.

Shifts in Relationships with Aging Parents: Many find themselves supporting elderly parents, managing the dual roles of caregiver and care recipient. This responsibility can create both stress and deeper family bonds, fostering a sense of mutual understanding.

Redefining Family Expectations and Boundaries: Individuals may feel a need to establish boundaries, especially around roles that no longer serve their well-being. Honest discussions can help clarify expectations, allowing family members to better support each other's evolving needs.

Evolving Social Roles and Self-Expression

As they re-evaluate social roles, individuals with disabilities often seek new communities and social circles that reflect their interests and aspirations.

Seeking New Social Identities: By exploring hobbies, spirituality, or advocacy groups, they connect with others who resonate with their current values, adding fulfilment to social interactions.

Distancing from Social Expectations: The confidence that comes with midlife can empower individuals to make choices that prioritize personal fulfilment over societal norms, creating a social life that feels truly meaningful.

Gender Differences in Midlife Crisis Symptoms for Persons with Disabilities

While midlife crises often involve universal themes of self-reflection and identity reassessment, experiences differ across gender and are further influenced by disability. Social conditioning, gender roles, and unique disability-related challenges shape how individuals confront midlife changes. Understanding these nuanced gendered experiences can provide valuable insight into how men and women with disabilities approach midlife, helping them navigate it with compassion, self-awareness, and resilience.

Midlife Crisis Symptoms in Men with Disabilities

For many men with disabilities, the midlife crisis centres around questions of career achievement, physical vitality, and societal roles. Men are often socialized to emphasize career success, physical strength, and financial security, but disability and aging may pose unique challenges to fulfilling these expectations. Common symptoms in men include:

Career Re-evaluation and Professional Discontent

For men with disabilities, professional achievements can be both a source of pride and frustration, especially if they have faced barriers related to accessibility or discrimination. During midlife, they may confront unfulfilled career ambitions or frustrations with their professional path, perhaps influenced by societal expectations or personal limitations. Some men may contemplate new careers or entrepreneurial ventures that allow more flexibility, while others may feel a renewed drive to make a significant impact in their field.

Physical Appearance and Health Concerns

Physical health and appearance concerns often intensify during midlife, and for men with disabilities, this can be shaped by complex interactions between disability, aging, and masculinity. Renewed efforts to maintain physical vitality, such as exercise or lifestyle changes, may be influenced by a desire to defy stereotypes around disability and aging. Some may seek adaptive sports, while others focus on managing health conditions to maximize independence and vitality.

Impulse for Novelty and Adventure

The stereotype of a man buying a sports car or taking on risky hobbies in midlife can hold true, but for men with disabilities, the impulse for novelty often manifests differently. Many pursue activities that offer a renewed sense of freedom and self-expression, such as adaptive sports, accessible travel, or engaging in hobbies that defy physical or societal constraints. This drive for novelty reflects a desire to experience life beyond perceived limitations and to feel empowered in new ways.

Increased Focus on Material and Financial Security

Financial security and legacy concerns often heighten in midlife. Men with disabilities may face additional financial planning considerations, such as future care needs, adaptive equipment, or housing modifications. Some may prioritize investments to secure independence, while others focus on building a legacy that reflects their accomplishments. This drive for financial stability often reflects a desire to ensure security for themselves and their families while affirming their value.

Emotional Isolation and Difficulty Expressing Vulnerability

Societal expectations can make it difficult for men to openly discuss vulnerabilities, and for men with disabilities, these challenges are often compounded by stigma. Midlife can bring loneliness and frustration, especially if they feel pressure to appear strong despite physical or emotional challenges. Support from trusted friends, peer groups, or mental health professionals familiar with disability issues can provide a safe space for expressing vulnerabilities and navigating this transitional phase.

Midlife Crisis Symptoms in Women with Disabilities

Women with disabilities often experience midlife as a time to reclaim identity beyond family, caregiving, or roles defined by others. For many, midlife represents an opportunity to explore unfulfilled aspirations while confronting unique challenges associated with disability and aging. Common symptoms in women include:

Identity Beyond Family and Caregiving Roles

Many women with disabilities spend years balancing roles as caregivers, family members, or community advocates, often putting others' needs before their own. Midlife can prompt the question, "Who am I beyond these roles and responsibilities?" This period often brings a desire to reclaim personal aspirations, pursue new goals, and define an identity independent of caregiving or disability status. This may involve exploring hobbies, professional interests, or advocacy that honors their evolving sense of self.

Physical Changes and Self-Image

Physical changes related to aging and disability may bring added self-reflection for women. Hormonal shifts, changes in physical abilities, or intensified health conditions can impact self-image, especially amid societal pressures for women to maintain youthfulness and beauty. This period may challenge self-confidence but can also offer an opportunity for growth, as women learn to embrace changes with resilience, focusing on strength, adaptability, and self-compassion.

Desire for Independence and Self-Discovery

Many women with disabilities experience a renewed desire for independence and self-expression during midlife. This may involve redefining boundaries, investing in personal interests, or setting aside time for self-care after years of prioritizing others. For some, this journey includes gaining greater control over their living environment, exploring adaptive hobbies, or connecting with other women who share similar experiences.

Re-evaluation of Relationships and Intimacy

Midlife can be a period when women with disabilities reassess their relationships, whether they are familial, platonic, or romantic. They may seek deeper intimacy and understanding from partners or friends, re-examining relational dynamics that may no longer serve their well-being. This phase can lead to new or renewed connections with people who appreciate them beyond their disability, fostering emotional growth and support.

Emotional Resilience and a Focus on Inner Growth

Many women approach a midlife crisis with a focus on self-reflection, resilience, and personal development. Women with disabilities may turn to supportive practices like therapy, meditation, or disability-specific support groups to process their emotions and navigate existential questions. This inner focus allows for growth, helping them explore purpose and reimagine fulfilment in ways that celebrate their resilience and adaptability.

Key Differences and Overlapping Experiences for Men and Women with Disabilities

While men and women with disabilities often experience a midlife crisis differently, there are overlapping challenges, such as navigating societal expectations and addressing personal growth needs. However, their approaches often diverge:

External vs. Internal Changes

Men's midlife crises tend to manifest externally, with visible changes in career pursuits, lifestyle, or material interests. Women's experiences are often more introspective, centered on self-discovery, relational dynamics, and reclaiming identity outside of caregiving or family roles.

Focus on Achievement vs. Relationships

Men often prioritize career achievements or financial security, motivated by a desire for legacy and stability. Women tend to focus on relational fulfilment, self-worth, and the pursuit of autonomy, re-evaluating relationships and redefining personal aspirations.

Navigating Vulnerability and Support

Societal pressures often make it challenging for men to express vulnerability, particularly if they feel that disability has limited their perceived strength. In contrast, women may be more open to discussing their emotions and seeking support from others. This willingness to embrace vulnerability can foster resilience, helping women adapt more easily to the challenges of midlife.

Understanding these differences highlights that there is no singular experience of a midlife crisis, especially for people with disabilities. Each journey is shaped by gendered expectations, personal history, and the unique impact of disability. Both men and women share common goals in midlife: the pursuit of authentic relationships, meaningful change, and lives aligned with their true values. By acknowledging the complexities of gender and disability, individuals can navigate midlife transitions with greater empathy, self-awareness, and resilience

Reframing the Midlife Crisis as a Journey of Growth and Empowerment

While the term "crisis" implies urgency or disruption, for persons with disabilities, this period can become an empowering experience, an opportunity to address past choices, reengage with passions, or reimagine what fulfilment looks like going forward. By understanding that a midlife crisis is not simply a period of difficulty but one of transformation, individuals with disabilities can find new paths that honor both their past achievements and future potential.

This process may include:

- Reassessing Relationships and Support Systems: Midlife often prompts reflection on relationships, and persons with disabilities may reevaluate support networks, determining what's most beneficial and sustainable for the years ahead.

- Reclaiming Identity Beyond Disability: As individuals navigate midlife, the desire to be seen and valued for more than one's disability often becomes central, fostering new self-expression and pursuits.

- **Exploring Adaptive Paths to Fulfillment:** Embracing growth might involve exploring creative, adaptive ways to pursue personal and professional goals within the context of any physical limitations or health changes that arise.

A midlife crisis, then, is not just about grappling with one's past or fearing the future. For persons with disabilities, it's a time to draw upon the resilience, adaptability, and strength they've developed, transforming this phase into one of meaningful reinvention and empowered self-discovery.

Chapter 4: A Different Journey: How Midlife Crisis Unfolds for People with Disabilities

Understanding Midlife Crisis Through Different Lenses

The term "midlife crisis" conjures images of introspection, re-evaluation, and often dramatic life changes. For many, midlife marks a significant turning point characterized by a mix of emotions and self-reflection as they reassess the meaning and purpose of their lives. Traditionally, a midlife crisis involves common themes: questioning career achievements, navigating shifting family dynamics, experiencing physical aging, and confronting unfulfilled dreams. However, while the experience of a midlife crisis differs vastly depending on personal background, health, and life experiences.

For individuals with disabilities, the midlife crisis takes on a unique dimension. The common themes remain present, but they are interwoven with additional layers of complexity, such as managing long-term health conditions, overcoming accessibility barriers, and dealing with societal perceptions of disability. These added factors create distinct challenges that can amplify or reshape the experience of midlife. This chapter explores these contrasts, shedding light on the ways a midlife crisis may differ for people with disabilities and highlighting the strength, resilience, and adaptability they often bring to this transitional period.

Unique Life Stages and Milestones

The path through life for people with disabilities often includes milestones and life stages that differ from the experiences of their non-disabled peers. Traditional markers of midlife, such as career achievements, retirement planning, and personal milestones like marriage or homeownership, may not follow the same trajectory for people with disabilities. Many individuals with disabilities face systemic barriers that impact their ability to reach these societal benchmarks.

For instance, educational and employment opportunities may be limited due to accessibility issues or discriminatory hiring practices, affecting career progression and financial independence. Social expectations around marriage, parenting, or independence can also create pressure, as many people with disabilities feel they are expected to adhere to societal standards that may not be achievable or desirable for them. These disparities can contribute to a sense of unfulfillment or frustration during midlife, particularly when reflecting on past goals or envisioning the future.

In contrast, non-disabled individuals often experience midlife as a time to evaluate their achievements within the context of these societal milestones, reflecting on their careers, relationships, and financial standing. For people with disabilities, however, midlife may highlight the differences between what they were able to achieve and what society typically expects, creating a unique dynamic in their midlife experience.

Health-Related Challenges in Midlife

Health plays a pivotal role in shaping the midlife experiences of people with disabilities. While midlife brings physical changes for most people, individuals with disabilities often face additional health considerations, which can significantly impact their experience. Many disabilities involve ongoing or progressive conditions, which may intensify as the body ages. This may require adjustments in treatment, increased medical support, or even changes to one's lifestyle that can further complicate the experience of midlife.

For instance, a person with a progressive condition, such as multiple sclerosis or muscular dystrophy, may face accelerated physical challenges as they age, heightening their anxiety about independence, mobility, and access to care. The constant management of health needs can limit the time and energy available for self-reflection or pursuing new passions during midlife, and the focus may instead shift to preserving quality of life.

Non-disabled individuals, on the other hand, may experience midlife as primarily a psychological shift, grappling with concepts of aging and mortality in a broader sense. While health concerns are often a component of midlife for everyone, for people with disabilities, these concerns may be more immediate and complex, shaping their midlife journey in ways that go beyond psychological reflection.

Identity and Societal Perception

For people with disabilities, midlife can bring about complex reflections on identity and self-worth, influenced by societal perceptions of disability. People with disabilities are often defined by others primarily in terms of their disability, and this societal labelling can impact their sense of identity. As they reach midlife, individuals may grapple with the desire to see themselves beyond this single dimension, searching for aspects of identity that reflect their passions, experiences, and unique personality rather than their disability alone.

However, societal biases and stereotypes can make this exploration challenging. While non-disabled individuals often grapple with issues of identity related to their accomplishments, relationships, or changing social roles, people with disabilities may feel the need to confront the limitations that others impose upon their identity. This can create a sense of conflict between how they perceive themselves and how society views them, which can be particularly pressing at midlife when the desire for a broader self-identity may feel urgent.

Midlife can become a period of introspection where individuals with disabilities seek to reclaim their narrative, working to redefine themselves in ways that feel authentic and empowering. This journey of self-definition is often more complex for people with disabilities than for their non-disabled peers, who may not face the same degree of external pressure on their identity.

Relationships and Social Isolation

Midlife is a period when relationships are often reassessed, and for people with disabilities, this can bring unique challenges. Social and romantic connections may be harder to form or maintain due to accessibility barriers, societal stigma, or physical limitations. People with disabilities might face additional scrutiny regarding their relationship status or independence, which can heighten feelings of isolation during midlife.

While non-disabled individuals may experience midlife as a time to seek new social connections or redefine relationships, individuals with disabilities may confront the reality of enduring social isolation. For some, physical limitations or the need for accessible environments make it difficult to participate in social gatherings or build connections, while others may face societal biases that make romantic relationships challenging to establish or maintain. This social isolation can amplify feelings of loneliness during midlife, making it a particularly sensitive period for people with disabilities.

The midlife crisis for people with disabilities often includes navigating these relationship dynamics, finding supportive communities, and fostering connections that provide understanding and companionship. For many, these relationships become an anchor, offering support through the complexities of midlife.

Employment, Financial Stability, and Career Satisfaction

Career and financial stability are central themes in midlife for many people, and they take on unique dimensions for those with disabilities. People with disabilities frequently encounter barriers in the workplace, from physical inaccessibility to discriminatory hiring practices, which can limit their career growth. These challenges are particularly significant at midlife, when people naturally reflect on their professional achievements and consider the financial security needed for later life.

Financial instability is a common stressor for people with disabilities, as employment gaps, limited access to high-paying positions, or reliance on disability benefits may create constraints. The struggle for meaningful work can feel amplified during midlife when societal pressure to "prove oneself" professionally may conflict with the realities of the job market for people with disabilities.

"I've been deaf since birth, and while I've held a steady job for years, I always felt limited in what I could achieve. In my late 40s, I tried to apply for a promotion, but they made it clear that 'communication challenges' were an issue. I realized then how precarious my position is. Without that promotion, I'm stuck with a lower salary, and insurance barely covers my healthcare needs. Lately, I've been working with a career coach who's helping me explore other job paths, and I'm building my confidence to try something new though the process is very slow." Priya, 50, Workplace discrimination.

For non-disabled individuals, midlife career challenges often involve evaluating one's position within a chosen field or contemplating retirement planning. For people with disabilities, however, midlife may reveal the impacts of systemic barriers, making it a time to navigate new financial strategies, seek out support networks, and redefine personal success beyond conventional career milestones.

Resilience, Adaptation, and Community Support

One of the defining features of midlife for people with disabilities is the remarkable resilience and adaptability that many develop over time. Facing a range of physical, social, and emotional challenges, people with disabilities often build strong coping mechanisms and support networks that serve them well during this transitional period. Communities of support—whether from advocacy groups, peer networks, or online spaces—provide valuable connection points and a sense of shared experience.

Both disabled and non disabled communities can act as both a resource and a refuge, providing practical advice, emotional support, and solidarity. While non-disabled individuals might seek conventional support systems, people with disabilities often find comfort in networks that understand their specific challenges, offering them strength and guidance through midlife.

Conclusion – Embracing a Unique Midlife Path

The midlife crisis for people with disabilities is marked by distinctive challenges and unique expressions of resilience. There are layered experiences that people with disabilities face, from health-related concerns to social isolation and career barriers. Despite these added complexities, individuals with disabilities navigate midlife with a resilience born from years of overcoming challenges, demonstrating adaptability and strength in the face of adversity.

This journey may differ from that of non-disabled individuals, but it is equally valid and deserves recognition. By understanding these differences, readers can develop a greater empathy and respect for the varied paths people with disabilities take during midlife. Ultimately, the midlife crisis for individuals with disabilities is a profound period of growth, reflection, and redefinition, filled with both struggles and triumphs.

Chapter 5: The Caregiver's Perspective

The Emotional and Physical Toll on Caregivers

Caregivers play a vital role in the lives of persons with disabilities, offering day-to-day support, emotional comfort, and often medical assistance. However, caregiving can be both physically and emotionally exhausting, especially when the person they care for is navigating a midlife crisis. During this time, the caregiver's responsibilities may increase as the individual's needs change due to the compounded effects of aging and disability.

Compassion Fatigue and Burnout: Supporting someone through a midlife crisis can lead to compassion fatigue, a state of emotional exhaustion from constantly providing empathy and support. Over time, this can lead to burnout, characterized by emotional depletion, physical fatigue, and a sense of detachment from the person they are caring for.

Emotional Exhaustion: Caregivers may feel overwhelmed by the ongoing emotional burden of comforting someone in the throes of their own emotional struggles.

Physical Exhaustion: The physical demands of caregiving—such as assisting with mobility, personal hygiene, or daily tasks—can strain the caregiver, especially if they are balancing caregiving with their own midlife challenges.

The Psychological Impact of Witnessing a Loved One's Struggle: Watching a loved one endure a midlife crisis can be deeply painful, especially when caregivers feel powerless to relieve their suffering. The person's feelings of regret, fear, or depression may resonate strongly with caregivers, adding to their emotional stress.

Feeling Helpless: Caregivers often wish they could do more but may feel helpless when emotional or psychological support seems insufficient.

Fear of the Future: Like the person they care for, caregivers may fear the future and worry about their ability to continue providing support, especially if their own health declines with age.

Balancing Caregiving with Personal Midlife Challenges

Caregivers may also be experiencing their own midlife transitions, and the emotional and physical toll of caregiving can amplify these personal struggles. Balancing their own midlife challenges with caregiving responsibilities can leave caregivers feeling overwhelmed and stretched thin.

The Caregiver's Own Midlife Crisis: Caregivers in midlife often face their own challenges, such as career changes, health, aging, financial concerns, or shifts in family roles. These personal stressors can make it harder to provide consistent emotional support to someone else.

"I've been taking care of my husband since his Parkinson's diagnosis seven years ago, and as the disease progresses, so do my responsibilities. I'm in my 50s now, and my own health is starting to show signs of wear—back pain, high blood pressure, constant fatigue. I barely have time for myself, and often feel torn between my own needs and his. Every day, I'm cooking special meals, managing his medications, and helping him with basic tasks, but there's no one to help me manage my own stress and health issues. We can't afford extra

---

Juggling Personal and Caregiving Responsibilities: Many caregivers must balance caregiving with other responsibilities, such as work and family obligations. This balancing act can create stress and guilt, as caregivers may feel they are not giving enough attention to any one area of their lives.

Guilt and Resentment: Caregivers commonly experience a mix of guilt and resentment, especially if their own needs are neglected or if the demands of caregiving become overwhelming.

Feeling Guilty for Needing a Break: Caregivers often feel guilty about needing personal time or expressing frustration, as they may believe they should be entirely devoted to the person they care for.

Resentment: Over time, caregivers may begin to feel resentment if they feel their lives are on hold. This feeling is more likely if they lack opportunities for respite or support.

Communicating and Supporting a Person in Crisis

A crucial aspect of caregiving during a midlife crisis is providing emotional support. This can be challenging, as the individual may experience intense emotional upheaval. However, open, compassionate communication is essential for helping them through the crisis.

Active Listening and Empathy: Caregivers can offer meaningful support by being active listeners and creating a safe space for the individual to express their feelings without fear of judgment. Practicing empathy and validating their emotions can be comforting, even when the conversations are difficult.

Avoiding Solutions-Based Responses: It's important for caregivers to resist the urge to "fix" the situation or offer immediate solutions. Often, the person in crisis simply needs to be heard and assured that their emotions are valid.

Recognizing the Signs of Crisis: Caregivers are often the first to notice signs of emotional distress, such as depression or anxiety. Recognizing these signals can help them provide the right support and seek professional help if needed.

Depression and Withdrawal: Signs like a lack of interest in activities, emotional numbness, or withdrawal from social interactions may indicate that the individual is struggling more than they are expressing.

Increased Dependence: If the individual starts relying more heavily on their caregiver for emotional or physical support, it may signal that they are overwhelmed by their crisis and may benefit from additional assistance.

Providing Emotional Support: Consistent emotional support is essential. Caregivers can help by being patient, encouraging open communication, and gently reminding the individual of their strengths and achievements.

Validating Their Feelings: Acknowledging the person's struggles without minimizing them is critical. Simple statements like "I can see this is really hard for you" or "It's okay to feel this way" can offer much-needed reassurance.

Balancing Caregiver and Personal Needs

It's essential for caregivers to remember that they cannot provide effective care if they neglect their own well-being. Self-care is not a luxury but a necessity for maintaining their own physical, emotional, and mental health.

Prioritizing Self-Care: Caregivers should make self-care a priority by scheduling regular breaks, seeking professional support for their own emotional needs, and setting boundaries to recharge.

Respite Care: Respite care offers temporary relief by allowing a professional or family member to step in. This enables caregivers to take necessary breaks and focus on their own well-being.

"My sister has been battling multiple sclerosis for over a decade, and as her condition has worsened, I've taken on the role of her primary caregiver. We live together, and while I work part-time to cover our living expenses, her medical needs often go beyond what I can afford. Every hospital visit, every new medicine—it all adds up.

Setting Boundaries: Establishing boundaries is essential for protecting caregivers' time and energy. This might involve designating specific times for personal activities or clearly communicating the need for help.

Communicating Boundaries: Caregivers should be clear about their boundaries with both the person they care for and other family members, explaining that personal time is essential for sustaining their caregiving responsibilities.

Seeking Support from Others: Caregiving doesn't have to be a solo effort. Building a support network—whether through friends, family, or professional resources—can help alleviate the sense of isolation that often accompanies caregiving.

Support Groups: Joining a caregiver support group provides an outlet for sharing experiences and solutions. Knowing that others face similar challenges can offer comfort and solidarity.

Building a Caregiver Support Network

Creating a strong support network is essential for caregivers to sustain their own well-being. This section explores how caregivers can establish a reliable circle of support, both professionally and personally.

Professional Support Services: Caregivers should take advantage of professional services like respite care, counselling, and financial or legal advisors. These resources can help reduce the stress of caregiving.

Caregiver Counselling: Talking with a therapist or counsellor specializing in caregiving issues can help caregivers process their emotions, manage stress, and protect their mental health.

Family and Friends: Reaching out to family and friends can provide both emotional relief and practical assistance. Having others occasionally help with caregiving tasks can ease the pressure on the primary caregiver.

Asking for Help: Many caregivers hesitate to ask for help, feeling they should manage everything independently. However, asking for support is essential for preventing burnout and ensuring they can continue providing effective care.

Online Communities and Resources: The internet provides a wealth of resources for caregivers, from online support groups to practical advice on self-care. Engaging with online communities can offer emotional support, especially for those who lack in-person options.

Finding Reliable Resources: It's important to seek out credible online resources, such as caregiver organizations or disability advocacy groups, which can provide accurate information and connect caregivers with helpful tools and support.

Chapter 6: Identity, Self-Worth, and Mental Health

Re-evaluating Self-Identity in Midlife

Midlife is a time of profound self-reflection, and for persons with disabilities, this stage brings unique challenges around identity and self-worth. Many individuals may have spent years adapting to and managing their condition, creating a sense of self deeply intertwined with their disability. However, as they approach midlife, shifting physical, emotional, and social dynamics may challenge and reshape this established identity.

Changes in Roles and Responsibilities: Many people define themselves by their roles—whether as professionals, parents, or caregivers. Midlife often prompts changes in these roles due to retirement, children becoming more independent, or evolving caregiving dynamics. For persons with disabilities, midlife may also mean increased reliance on others, which can bring feelings of loss or diminished purpose.

Impact of Societal Perceptions: Societal attitudes toward disability can significantly influence self-perception. In midlife, individuals may feel heightened societal pressure related to their appearance, abilities, or productivity, especially if they already feel marginalized due to their disability. Facing these external perceptions can be emotionally taxing and may challenge long-held beliefs about self-worth.

Psychological Aspects of the Midlife Crisis

A midlife crisis often brings psychological challenges, and these can be amplified for persons with disabilities. Recognizing the common psychological impacts during this stage is essential for fostering mental health and resilience.

Anxiety and Fear of the Future: Anxiety is common in midlife, often centred around aging, health concerns, and the uncertainty of the future. Persons with disabilities may experience this anxiety more intensely as they face questions about health, mobility, and independence in the years ahead.

Progressive Disabilities: Individuals with progressive conditions, such as multiple sclerosis, muscular dystrophy, or Parkinson's disease, may worry about how their illness will evolve and impact their quality of life.

Caregiver Concerns: Those reliant on caregivers may fear losing their primary support system if circumstances change. This worry can lead to persistent anxiety about future care needs and quality of life.

Depression and Emotional Strain: Depression is a common feature of the midlife crisis, often driven by feelings of unfulfilled potential, physical limitations, or social isolation. For persons with disabilities, who may have already faced depression earlier in life, these emotions may resurface or intensify in midlife.

Loss of Control and Helplessness: Midlife can bring a sense of loss, whether of independence, physical capabilities, or life opportunities. For persons with disabilities, this helplessness may deepen as their reliance on support increases.

Grieving Unmet Expectations: Midlife can also prompt grief for lost opportunities or unachieved dreams. This grief may feel especially poignant for those whose disability has influenced the direction of their lives in unforeseen ways.

Self-Esteem and Body Image: Physical aging often brings challenges around body image and self-esteem. For persons with disabilities, age-related physical changes may compound feelings of inadequacy or diminished self-worth.

Comparisons with Non-Disabled Peers: Comparisons to peers without disabilities can intensify feelings of frustration or inadequacy, as individuals may perceive themselves as limited by circumstances outside their control.

Changes in Physical Appearance: The visible signs of aging can be particularly difficult for those who have already experienced body changes due to their disability, creating compounded challenges around self-acceptance.

Managing Depression, Anxiety, and Emotional Strain

Addressing the psychological dimensions of the midlife crisis is essential for navigating this period with resilience. Several strategies and interventions can help individuals manage emotional strain and foster mental well-being.

Therapy and Counselling: Therapy is a valuable resource for those struggling with midlife emotional challenges, especially for persons with disabilities who may face compounded issues. Cognitive-behavioural therapy (CBT) can help individuals reframe negative thought patterns and build effective coping strategies.

Grief Counselling: Counselling that focuses on grieving lost opportunities or physical abilities can support emotional healing and acceptance.

Support Groups: Participating in support groups—whether for individuals with disabilities or those navigating midlife—can alleviate feelings of isolation. Group settings provide a space to share experiences and receive support from others facing similar challenges.

Mindfulness and Stress Management Techniques: Mindfulness-based stress reduction (MBSR) and similar techniques can be effective for managing midlife anxiety and depression. By focusing on the present, individuals can reduce worry about the future and regret about the past.

Meditation and Relaxation Exercises: Practices like meditation and deep breathing can reduce stress and promote balance, helping individuals feel more connected to their bodies despite physical limitations.

Journaling and Reflection: Journaling can provide a therapeutic outlet for processing difficult emotions. Writing about fears, regrets, or hopes can help individuals gain perspective and move forward with greater clarity.

Medication and Mental Health Support: In cases of severe depression or anxiety, medication may be necessary. Consulting with a healthcare professional to explore treatment options is an important step in managing mental health during midlife.

Building Self-Worth and Personal Growth

Despite the challenges of midlife, this phase also offers opportunities for personal growth and a redefinition of self-worth. With the right support and strategies, individuals can emerge from this stage with renewed purpose and a strengthened sense of identity.

"I was diagnosed with dyslexia as a kid, and while I developed coping strategies, I've always felt like an imposter at work, constantly afraid I'll slip up. Now, hitting my late 40s, I started wondering if I've reached my ceiling. But after talking to a friend, I decided to open up to my boss and team about my challenges. Turns out, they're incredibly supportive, and I'm now taking the lead on projects that play to my strengths. Embracing my disability instead of hiding it has been

---

Redefining Success and Achievement: Redefining what success and fulfilment look like can be transformative. For persons with disabilities, this may involve moving away from traditional markers of success (such as career achievements or financial milestones) and focusing instead on more personal, meaningful goals (such as relationships, personal growth, or community contributions).

Focusing on Areas of Control: Instead of dwelling on areas of life that feel out of control, individuals can focus on aspects where they still have agency. This might include pursuing hobbies, advocating for themselves in healthcare settings, or engaging in support or advocacy groups.

"Losing my sight felt like losing myself. I'd built my life around my work as a photographer, and now I'm legally blind. What am I if I can't capture the world around me? It took years of counselling to realize I'm still me, still creative. Now, I'm exploring audio storytelling, creating art that taps into sound. It's different, sure, but it's given me a purpose again. I may not be able to see my work,

but I can still create something that others can feel." Sameer 42, Vision loss and identity crisis

---

Celebrating Small Wins: Acknowledging small achievements—whether managing daily tasks, setting and achieving personal goals, or maintaining independence—can help rebuild self-worth. Each accomplishment can serve as a stepping stone toward greater confidence and purpose.

Embracing Change: Instead of resisting midlife changes, individuals can benefit from embracing them as part of their growth. This might mean adapting to new caregiving arrangements or finding creative ways to engage in meaningful activities. Acceptance can foster a healthier emotional outlook.

Mental Health Resources and Therapeutic Interventions

Accessing the right resources and therapeutic interventions is crucial for managing the psychological challenges of the midlife crisis. Mental health professionals and healthcare providers offer a range of services to support individuals through this transition.

Therapeutic Approaches: Depending on the individual's needs, various therapeutic approaches, including cognitive-behavioral therapy (CBT), dialectical behaviour therapy (DBT), and mindfulness-based therapies, can provide valuable tools for managing emotions and building resilience.

Finding the Right Professional: It is essential for individuals to find a mental health professional who understands the complexities of the midlife crisis and is experienced in working with persons with disabilities. Tailored mental health care can address the unique challenges of this period effectively.

Chapter 7: Relationships, Family, and Social Dynamics

Impact on Personal and Romantic Relationships

Midlife often marks a period of transition for personal and romantic relationships, and for persons with disabilities, these shifts can bring additional complexities. The evolving physical, emotional, and psychological landscape of midlife affects both established and new relationships in unique ways.

Disability-Specific Challenges in Romantic Relationships: Disabilities can introduce unique challenges to romantic relationships, particularly during midlife. For individuals who acquired a disability later in life, navigating midlife may involve adjusting to new limitations that alter the relationship dynamic.

Mobility Disabilities: Individuals with mobility impairments may face increased physical challenges in midlife, such as reduced stamina or chronic pain, which can affect physical intimacy and the way couples connect. Exploring new forms of intimacy and communication can help couples adapt to these changes.

Neurological Disabilities: When one partner experiences cognitive decline, such as early-onset dementia or progressive conditions like Parkinson's disease, maintaining an emotional connection can become difficult. The caregiving role often intensifies, which may strain the romantic aspect of the relationship.

Sensory Disabilities: For individuals who are deaf, hard of hearing, or blind, midlife may bring additional communication challenges, especially as their partner faces age-related changes. Couples may need to find new ways to communicate effectively as hearing or vision declines.

Navigating Changing Dynamics: In long-term relationships, midlife often brings a re-evaluation of roles and responsibilities. For persons with disabilities, this period may coincide with increasing caregiving needs, which can place stress on the partnership.

Balancing Caregiving and Partnership: As caregiving responsibilities grow, partners may struggle to balance the roles of caregiver and romantic partner. Open communication about how these changes impact the relationship and seeking outside support when needed can help maintain a healthy dynamic.

Sexual Intimacy and Aging with a Disability: Sexuality and intimacy can be particularly complex in midlife, especially for individuals with disabilities. Changes in physical ability, body image, and libido may affect sexual relationships. Finding adaptive solutions can help couples maintain physical closeness and intimacy despite these changes.

Family Dynamics and Support Systems

Midlife often brings significant changes within family structures. For persons with disabilities, this period may involve renegotiating family relationships, especially regarding caregiving and support.

The Role of Family Caregivers: Family members frequently assume caregiving roles, either gradually over time or more abruptly as needs increase. In midlife, caregiving dynamics may shift, especially as disabilities become more complex with age.

Chronic Illnesses and Progressive Disabilities: Individuals with chronic or progressive conditions like multiple sclerosis or muscular dystrophy may require increasing levels of care from family members as they age. This can place additional strain on familial relationships, especially when caregivers must balance these duties with their own midlife challenges.

Intergenerational Caregiving: Midlife may also involve caring for aging parents, even while receiving care themselves. This intergenerational caregiving dynamic can be emotionally taxing, particularly if external support systems are limited.

Parenting with a Disability in Midlife: Many individuals with disabilities are parents, and navigating midlife can involve balancing personal changes with parenting responsibilities. This can be challenging when disabilities affect the ability to engage in day-to-day parenting activities.

Disability-Specific Parenting Challenges: Parents with mobility disabilities may find it increasingly difficult to participate in activities with their children as they age. Similarly, parents with sensory disabilities may face communication challenges if their condition worsens during midlife.

Explaining Disability and Midlife Changes to Children: Parents with disabilities may need to explain both their disability and the changes that come with midlife to their children, which can be challenging if children struggle to understand why their parent's abilities are changing.

"I've dealt with chronic pain since my late 30s, and it's been especially tough raising two teenagers. Sometimes, I feel like I'm letting them down because I can't keep up with their activities or be the active mom I always wanted to be. But lately, I've started focusing on what I can do—long talks, helping with homework, and just being there for them emotionally. I joined an online group of moms with disabilities, and we swap ideas on how to be present in our kids' lives. I'm learning to give myself grace and redefine what being a good mom means." Nina, 49, with chronic pain difficulties

---

Sibling and Extended Family Relationships: Midlife may also bring shifts in relationships with siblings and extended family members. For persons with disabilities, these relationships may be affected by caregiving expectations, financial pressures, or differing views on the best way to provide support.

Varying Levels of Support: Family members may have different capacities to provide care or emotional support. While some may step up to help, others may find it difficult to balance their own responsibilities with caregiving, which can lead to tension.

Expanding Social Networks

Social relationships are an important source of support and connection during midlife, but for persons with disabilities, building and maintaining social networks can be challenging. Physical limitations, societal stigma, and inaccessible environments can all create barriers to forming and sustaining friendships.

The Impact of Isolation: Many persons with disabilities experience social isolation, which can worsen during midlife. Isolation can lead to feelings of loneliness, depression, and decreased self-worth, especially if individuals can no longer participate in activities they once enjoyed.

Mobility and Access Challenges: For individuals with mobility impairments, physical access to social spaces may become more difficult in midlife as stamina decreases or pain increases. Transportation barriers, inaccessible venues, and limited opportunities for social engagement can contribute to isolation.

Communication Barriers: Those with sensory disabilities may encounter additional communication barriers that make socializing challenging, particularly if hearing or vision further declines. For example, individuals who are deaf may face fewer social opportunities if they rely on interpreters or if friends are less willing to accommodate their communication needs.

Building New Social Connections: Expanding social networks during midlife is crucial for emotional well-being. For persons with disabilities, finding new social outlets might involve joining disability-specific support groups or participating in accessible community activities.

Disability-Specific Social Groups: Many communities have support groups or social organizations for individuals with disabilities. These groups offer not only social engagement but also emotional support from peers facing similar midlife challenges. Mei, 50 - Hearing Loss and Relationship Strain

Online Communities and Social Media: For those who have difficulty accessing physical social spaces, online communities can provide a meaningful way to stay connected. Social media platforms, forums, and virtual support groups allow individuals with disabilities to build relationships and share experiences with others who understand their challenges.

Navigating Relationship Stigmas and Societal Expectations

Societal perceptions of disability can often influence how individuals are treated in their relationships, both personal and social. Midlife may bring renewed attention to societal expectations, particularly concerning relationships, body image, and independence.

Stigmas Surrounding Disability and Relationships: Society often holds preconceived notions about the romantic and sexual lives of persons with disabilities. These stigmas can add emotional strain for individuals who are already navigating the challenges of midlife.

Sexuality and Disability: Society may wrongly assume that persons with disabilities are less interested in or capable of engaging in romantic or sexual relationships. This stigma can lead to feelings of inadequacy or frustration, particularly for those dealing with bodily changes in midlife.

Body Image and Confidence: Body image concerns commonly arise during midlife, and for persons with disabilities, these concerns may be amplified by societal judgments about physical appearance and ability. Individuals may feel pressured to conform to unrealistic beauty standards, which can negatively affect self-worth.

Overcoming External Expectations: Breaking free from societal expectations about disability and midlife involves developing a strong sense of self and building a supportive community that values individuality beyond societal norms.

Challenging Stereotypes: Persons with disabilities, along with their partners and families, can challenge stereotypes by advocating for better representation in media, participating in activism, or sharing personal experiences to promote a broader understanding of disability in midlife.

Educating Others: In some cases, individuals may need to educate their social circles about the realities of living with a disability during midlife. Open conversations can help reduce stigma and create a more supportive environment for both personal and social relationships.

"Living with multiple sclerosis isn't visible to most people, and I've always felt I had to downplay it. In my 50s now, it feels like no one quite understands what I'm going through, even family members. Lately, I've started volunteering at a support group, and sharing my story has been surprisingly therapeutic. It's helped me reconnect with others and feel part of a community that gets it. I don't have to explain myself there, and that has been a lifeline as I redefine who I am in this new phase of

life." Komal. 50, Multiple sclerosis and social isolation.

life." Komal. 50, Multiple sclerosis and social isolation.

Chapter 8: Career, Finances, and Retirement Planning

Managing Career Changes

Midlife often prompts people to reconsider their career paths or make significant changes in their professional lives. For persons with disabilities, navigating career transitions can be particularly complex, as disabilities may impact work performance, mobility, or energy levels. This section examines disability-specific career challenges and strategies for adapting to these changes.

Disability-Specific Career Challenges:

Mobility Disabilities: Individuals with mobility impairments, such as those who use wheelchairs or have conditions like cerebral palsy or spinal cord injuries, may face increased physical challenges in midlife, affecting their ability to continue in physically demanding jobs. Shifting to more sedentary roles or remote work can help them stay engaged professionally.

Example: A person with a spinal cord injury working in construction management may find that midlife brings increased pain or fatigue.

Transitioning to a desk-based role, such as project planning or consultancy, allows them to continue contributing while adapting to their physical needs.

"I never thought I'd still be in the same role after two decades, but here I am. I always wanted to move up in my career, but after my accident in my late 30s, everything slowed down. Navigating the office in a wheelchair made me feel like an outsider, and people started treating me differently. I felt stuck—both literally and figuratively. But recently, I found a mentor who's also a wheelchair user. He's shown me it's possible to lead and inspire from wherever you are. I'm rethinking my path, aiming for leadership roles, and finally feel I have a shot at something more." Jatin, 47, Mobility Impairment and Career Challenges

---

Cognitive Disabilities: Individuals with cognitive disabilities or progressive neurological conditions, like early-onset dementia or multiple sclerosis, may face increased difficulties with focus and memory, which can affect their ability to perform in fast-paced environments. They may benefit from accommodations or considering early retirement.

Example: A professional with multiple sclerosis may struggle with concentration and memory lapses in a high-pressure role. Shifting to part-time work or a slower-paced position can allow them to remain professionally engaged while managing cognitive changes.

Sensory Disabilities: Individuals who are blind, deaf, or hard of hearing may find it challenging to navigate careers in environments primarily designed for non-disabled individuals. As they age, additional accommodations may be required to support effective communication and performance.

Example: A public relations professional who is deaf might face greater communication barriers as their hearing declines with age. Transitioning to a role focused on written communication, like digital content creation, can help them remain productive and connected.

Career Flexibility and Adaptive Work Environments: Persons with disabilities can thrive in their careers by adapting their work environments or exploring new roles that align with their evolving needs. Many employers are increasingly supportive of workplace accommodations, and technological advances make it easier for individuals to work into midlife.

Remote Work Opportunities: The rise of remote work offers greater flexibility, particularly beneficial for those with mobility or sensory impairments. Working from home allows individuals to set up accessible environments and avoid commuting challenges.

Adaptive Technology: Advances in technology, such as screen readers, voice recognition software, and other assistive devices, enable individuals with disabilities to work effectively and adapt to changing physical or sensory needs.

Financial Planning for Midlife with Disabilities

Financial planning is crucial for everyone in midlife, but persons with disabilities may face additional costs related to medical needs, assistive devices, and long-term care. This section addresses key financial considerations and strategies for building resilience.

Disability-Specific Financial Considerations:

Medical Expenses: Many individuals with disabilities face higher medical costs in midlife, particularly if their condition requires ongoing treatment, medication, or surgeries. These expenses may not be fully covered by insurance, leading to financial strain.

Example: An individual with a degenerative condition, like muscular dystrophy, may need more frequent medical care or new assistive devices as they age, increasing out-of-pocket costs.

Assistive Technology and Home Modifications: As physical needs change, individuals may require new assistive technology or home modifications, such as stairlifts, adjustable beds, or specialized mobility devices.

Example: A person with cerebral palsy may find that their current wheelchair no longer meets their needs as they age. Upgrading to a custom-built chair and making home modifications, like widening doorways, can add to financial pressure.

Caregiving Costs: Midlife may bring the need for professional caregiving services, from part-time assistance with daily tasks to full-time in-home care, depending on the severity of the disability.

Example: An individual with advanced multiple sclerosis might need to hire a caregiver for help with personal hygiene, mobility, and household tasks, adding a significant financial burden alongside ongoing medical expenses.

Building Financial Resilience:

Disability Benefits and Government Assistance: In India, many individuals with disabilities rely on various government programs and schemes to help manage living and medical expenses. Key programs include the Disability Pension provided by state governments, the Indira Gandhi National Disability Pension Scheme (IGNDPS) under the National Social Assistance Programme (NSAP), and subsidies for assistive devices under schemes like the Assistance to Disabled Persons for Purchase/Fitting of Aids and Appliances (ADIP) scheme. Understanding eligibility criteria and maximizing these benefits is essential for financial stability.

Navigating the Benefits System: The process of applying for and accessing disability benefits in India can be complex, often involving multiple levels of bureaucracy. Working with financial advisors or social workers who are familiar with disability support schemes can help ensure individuals receive the benefits they are entitled to. Additionally, connecting with NGOs and disability advocacy groups can provide guidance and support in navigating government assistance programs.

Navigating the Benefits System: Applying for and maintaining disability benefits can be complex. Working with financial advisors or legal professionals can help ensure individuals receive the full benefits they're entitled to.

Long-Term Financial Planning: Effective financial planning for midlife includes provisions for long-term care, retirement, and potential medical costs. Savings, investments, and insurance policies can provide stability and security for the future.

Example: A person with a mobility disability might work with a financial planner to set aside funds for future caregiving, home modifications, and medical needs, with long-term care insurance as an added safeguard.

Planning for Retirement with a Disability

Retirement planning is a priority in midlife, and for persons with disabilities, it comes with additional considerations. This section covers disability-specific retirement planning, including when to retire, managing healthcare costs, and strategies for financial independence.

Disability-Specific Retirement Challenges:

Early Retirement Due to Health Decline: Some individuals with disabilities experience worsening symptoms in midlife, making early retirement a necessary option. Planning for the financial implications of retiring early is crucial.

Example: A person with Parkinson's disease experiencing rapid progression in their 50s may need to retire sooner than planned. This requires adjusting financial goals to account for a longer reliance on savings and benefits.

Healthcare Costs in Retirement: Managing healthcare costs is a major concern for individuals with disabilities in retirement. Medicare, Medicaid, and private insurance may cover some expenses, but out-of-pocket costs for long-term care, medical equipment, and medications are likely.

Example: A retired person with ALS (amyotrophic lateral sclerosis) may require extensive home care, specialized equipment, and ongoing treatments. Understanding coverage and preparing for out-of-pocket costs is essential for financial stability in retirement.

Maintaining Financial Independence in Retirement: Financial independence is essential to a good quality of life in retirement. Persons with disabilities can take proactive steps in midlife to secure their future and reduce reliance on family or public assistance.

Savings and Investment Strategies: Building a retirement fund is key, and it's important to consider the specific costs associated with a disability. Consulting with a financial advisor who understands disability planning can help in creating a retirement strategy that includes medical and caregiving expenses.

Example: A person with a visual impairment may allocate savings for assistive technology upgrades, like screen readers or Braille devices, to ensure they remain functional and independent throughout retirement.

Social Security and Disability Benefits: Understanding how Social Security retirement benefits interact with disability payments is essential for maximizing income in retirement.

Example: An individual with a spinal cord injury who receives SSDI may need guidance on transitioning to Social Security retirement benefits to ensure a smooth transition and maximize available income.

Balancing Financial Security with Quality of Life

While financial planning is essential, it's also important for individuals to balance financial goals with quality of life. Midlife is a time for many people to reevaluate priorities, and for persons with disabilities, this may mean choosing fulfilment over financial gain.

Pursuing New Passions in Midlife: Midlife may offer an opportunity to explore passions or hobbies that were previously set aside. This might involve a career change, reduced work hours, or investing in meaningful personal pursuits.

Example: A person with a hearing impairment who previously worked in a corporate environment may choose to retire early and start a small art business, finding fulfillment in a creative field rather than focusing solely on financial stability.

Financial Support for Personal Goals: Financial planning in midlife should include resources for personal well-being, whether for travel, education, or adaptive hobbies that bring joy and satisfaction.

Example: An individual with a mobility disability might allocate part of their retirement savings toward accessible travel, ensuring that retirement years are not only financially secure but also personally rewarding.

Chapter 9: Physical Health Concerns in Midlife for Persons with Disabilities

Understanding the Intersection of Aging, Disability, and Physical Health

As individuals age, their bodies naturally undergo changes. For persons with disabilities, these changes can be more pronounced or may occur earlier. Disabilities can accelerate the aging process, exacerbate existing health conditions, and increase susceptibility to new physical challenges. This section explores the intersection of disabilities and aging, highlighting specific health concerns that arise during midlife.

Aging and Accelerated Decline: Individuals with disabilities often face age-related health issues sooner than their non-disabled peers. This can include joint pain, muscle weakness, and reduced mobility. For instance, individuals with physical disabilities may experience more rapid declines in muscle mass and may encounter chronic pain earlier than others.

Example: A person with cerebral palsy may develop increased muscle stiffness and joint pain by their 40s, whereas their non-disabled peers might encounter these issues later in life. This accelerated decline may necessitate more frequent medical interventions or physical therapy.

Cumulative Effects of Long-Term Disabilities: Individuals who have lived with disabilities for years often face additional physical issues in midlife due to the cumulative effects of their condition. Repeated strain on specific body parts, overuse injuries, and prolonged immobility can contribute to issues such as joint deterioration or cardiovascular complications.

Example: A person who has used a wheelchair for decades may develop shoulder or wrist pain from years of overuse, making it harder to maintain independence in daily tasks.

Compounded Health Risks: Disabilities can increase the risk of conditions like cardiovascular disease, diabetes, and osteoporosis. These risks can be compounded by aging, requiring individuals to adopt a proactive approach to health and preventive care.

Example: A person with a spinal cord injury might face a heightened risk of cardiovascular issues due to reduced mobility, and this risk often increases with age.

How Different Disabilities Can Increase the Likelihood of Health Conditions

Certain disabilities heighten the likelihood of developing specific health issues in midlife. Understanding these risks is essential for proactive health management and timely medical intervention. Below, we examine common health concerns associated with various types of disabilities.

Mobility Disabilities: Individuals with mobility impairments, such as those with spinal cord injuries, multiple sclerosis, or muscular dystrophy, are at higher risk for musculoskeletal issues, joint degeneration, and cardiovascular disease.

Musculoskeletal Issues: Long-term reliance on assistive devices or overcompensation by certain muscle groups can lead to musculoskeletal problems like joint deterioration, arthritis, or chronic pain.

Example: A person using a wheelchair may develop shoulder pain from years of transferring or self-propelling. Over time, this can result in degenerative joint issues requiring medical intervention.

Cardiovascular Disease: Reduced mobility often leads to a sedentary lifestyle, increasing the risk of cardiovascular disease. Individuals with limited mobility should prioritize regular cardiovascular check-ups to monitor heart health.

Sensory Disabilities: Individuals who are blind, have low vision, or are deaf face unique physical challenges as they age. Lack of certain senses may increase the risk of accidents, falls, and musculoskeletal strain due to overcompensation.

Fall Risks: Vision impairments can increase the likelihood of falls, which can lead to fractures or other injuries. Aging further heightens the risk due to decreased bone density and slower recovery times.

Example: A person with low vision may face challenges with balance and coordination, increasing the risk of falls, particularly in unfamiliar environments or spaces lacking visual cues.

Overcompensation Injuries: Relying on certain body parts or senses to compensate for a disability can lead to strain injuries, such as neck or back pain. For example, individuals who are deaf may rely heavily on vision, leading to eye strain or neck discomfort from frequently turning to face speakers.

Neurological Disabilities: Neurological conditions, such as cerebral palsy, Parkinson's disease, or epilepsy, often increase the risk of additional health issues as the body ages. These conditions frequently come with progressive physical and cognitive decline that requires regular medical management.

Progressive Decline: Neurological conditions may worsen over time, leading to greater mobility challenges, coordination issues, and cognitive impairments. Individuals with these conditions need consistent medical support to manage symptoms and prevent complications.

Example: A person with Parkinson's disease might experience increased tremors, muscle stiffness, and walking difficulties as they age, necessitating adjustments to their treatment and physical therapy.

Respiratory and Cardiovascular Issues: Neurological disabilities can heighten the risk of respiratory infections, pneumonia, and cardiovascular problems, particularly for individuals with limited mobility or exercise capacity.

Medical Check-Ups and Screenings: A Proactive Approach

Proactive healthcare is essential for managing midlife health risks associated with disabilities. Regular check-ups and targeted screenings allow early detection and timely care, helping individuals maintain their health and independence. Below are some recommended check-ups and screenings for persons with disabilities in midlife.

General Health Check-Ups

Annual Physical Exams: Routine physical exams are vital for monitoring overall health and addressing emerging concerns. The checklist of the essential examinations is given in the appendix of the book.

Bone Density Scans: Bone density scans are important for identifying osteoporosis, especially in individuals with limited mobility. Early detection can help prevent fractures and promote bone health.

Example: A person with a spinal cord injury should undergo regular bone density tests, as reduced weight-bearing activity raises the risk of bone loss.

Specialized Check-Ups Based on Disability

Cardiovascular Health: Individuals with mobility impairments or sedentary lifestyles should undergo regular cardiovascular screenings, such as EKGs and stress tests, to monitor heart health. Engaging in modified forms of exercise is also beneficial for cardiovascular fitness.

Example: A person with muscular dystrophy should have regular heart screenings, as their condition can impact the heart muscles and lead to cardiomyopathy or other issues.

Joint Health and Musculoskeletal Assessments: Regular assessments for joint health are crucial for individuals with mobility disabilities. X-rays, MRIs, or physical therapy evaluations can help detect joint degeneration or musculoskeletal problems early.

Example: A person who uses crutches or a wheelchair may benefit from annual assessments to identify signs of overuse injuries or joint deterioration.

Cancer Screenings

Aging individuals with disabilities may face a higher risk for certain cancers due to lifestyle, genetic factors, or long-term medication use. Regular screenings, such as mammograms, colonoscopies, and skin cancer checks, are essential for early detection.

Example: A woman with limited mobility may face difficulties in accessing regular mammograms due to accessibility issues. Ensuring healthcare facilities are accessible is crucial to prevent missed screenings.

Neurological and Cognitive Health Assessments

Individuals with neurological conditions should have regular cognitive health assessments to monitor for early signs of dementia, Alzheimer's, or other cognitive impairments. Brain scans, cognitive tests, and neurological exams can help detect issues early.

Example: A person with epilepsy may experience cognitive decline over time, making regular check-ups with a neurologist important for monitoring brain function and adjusting medications as necessary.

Preventive Health and Lifestyle Adjustments

Alongside medical check-ups, preventive health strategies are crucial for promoting well-being and preventing future complications. Lifestyle adjustments—such as a balanced diet, regular physical activity, and stress management—play a key role.

Nutrition and Diet: Proper nutrition supports energy levels, immune function, and chronic disease prevention. Persons with disabilities may benefit from working with a nutritionist to develop a diet that aligns with their specific health needs.

Example: A person with limited mobility may require a low-calorie, nutrient-dense diet to prevent weight gain and support cardiovascular health, while someone with gastrointestinal issues might avoid certain foods that trigger discomfort.

Adaptive Exercise Programs: Physical activity helps maintain muscle strength, flexibility, and cardiovascular health, but traditional exercise routines may need adjustments for persons with disabilities. Working with a physical therapist to create a tailored program can help individuals stay active.

Example: A person with a mobility disability might engage in seated exercises or water therapy to stay fit, while someone with arthritis could benefit from low-impact activities like swimming or yoga.

"After losing my leg in my 30s, I worked hard to stay active. But now, with age, even simple tasks seem to take twice as much energy. I miss the athlete I used to be and sometimes feel defeated by my body. But I recently joined a local adaptive sports team, and training with others who understand the struggle has been a game-changer. I'm not as fast as I used to be, but I'm still in the game. It feels great to belong to a team again." Omar, 51, Amputation and physical fitness

---

Mental Health and Stress Management: The emotional challenges of midlife, combined with the physical demands of managing a disability, can increase stress, anxiety, and depression. Engaging in stress-reducing practices like mindfulness, meditation, or counselling can support mental well-being.

Example: A person experiencing chronic pain may benefit from mindfulness meditation to reduce the emotional toll of their condition, while regular counselling sessions can provide coping strategies for managing frustration or fear.

Chapter 10: Navigating the Healthcare System

The healthcare system is a crucial support for persons with disabilities, especially as they enter mid-life and encounter new or worsening physical and mental health challenges. Healthcare providers play an essential role in helping individuals navigate this critical stage, but the system can often feel overwhelming, both for persons with disabilities and their caregivers. From understanding the role of healthcare professionals to addressing access barriers, this chapter provides a comprehensive guide to creating a healthcare plan that supports both physical and emotional well-being.

The Role of Healthcare Professionals in Mid-Life Crisis Management

Healthcare providers must recognize the multifaceted nature of the mid-life crisis for persons with disabilities. Primary care physicians, specialists, and mental health practitioners have a unique responsibility to offer care that addresses physical symptoms as well as emotional and psychological needs.

Understanding the Emotional and Psychological Impact: Healthcare providers often focus primarily on managing the physical aspects of a disability. However, it's equally important for them to understand the emotional toll a mid-life crisis can impose. Conditions like anxiety, depression, or emotional withdrawal may develop, especially if the individual is struggling with changes in independence or self-identity. Healthcare professionals need to consider these factors as part of a holistic care plan.

Example: A person with a progressive condition like multiple sclerosis (MS) may experience anxiety about losing further mobility as they age. Routine appointments should include mental health screenings to detect signs of depression or anxiety early, ensuring that these issues are addressed alongside physical health.

Building a Collaborative Care Plan: A successful healthcare plan for mid-life individuals with disabilities should be multidisciplinary. This approach integrates primary care, specialty care, mental health support, and rehabilitative services, ensuring that each aspect of a person's health is addressed.

Holistic Care: Holistic care recognizes the interconnectedness of physical, mental, and emotional health. Providers should facilitate open conversations about emotional well-being, not just physical symptoms. Integrating therapy, support groups, or counseling into routine care can be especially beneficial for individuals dealing with the life transitions that mid-life brings.

Example: For someone with cerebral palsy, a collaborative plan might include a neurologist, a physical therapist, and a counsellor who specializes in disability. This team can address physical therapy needs, emotional support, and any emerging neurological symptoms.

Challenges in Healthcare Access for Mid-Life Persons with Disabilities

Navigating the healthcare system can be complex and frustrating for anyone, but persons with disabilities may face additional barriers. These barriers can stem from financial limitations, structural inadequacies, and insufficient disability-specific training among healthcare providers.

Financial Barriers and Insurance Issues: The cost of healthcare can be especially burdensome for persons with disabilities, who may need more frequent doctor visits, specialized treatments, and assistive devices as they age. For instance, a person with a spinal cord injury may require ongoing physical therapy to maintain mobility and prevent secondary complications. Lack of financial resources might force them to either reduce treatment or pay out of pocket, increasing financial strain.

Limited Insurance Coverage: Many insurance plans do not cover the full range of care that persons with disabilities need. Services like physical therapy, mental health counselling, or adaptive devices might be only partially covered or excluded altogether, placing a significant financial burden on individuals and their families.

"I rely on my monthly disability pension, but with the rising cost of living, it feels like I'm barely scraping by. My treatments for multiple sclerosis eat up a massive portion of my income, especially since physical therapy isn't covered under most affordable health insurance plans. Every new symptom means more consultations and tests, and I often ask myself if I can even afford to go to the doctor. I don't have access to any grants or

---

Navigating Bureaucracy: Managing insurance claims and paperwork can be time-consuming and overwhelming. Individuals with disabilities may require additional support to ensure they receive the benefits they are entitled to, especially under complex public assistance programs.

Example: Someone with a hearing impairment may face obstacles in obtaining coverage for cochlear implants or hearing aids due to restrictive insurance policies. Working with social workers or advocates can help navigate these bureaucratic hurdles.

Accessibility Issues in Healthcare Facilities: Physical barriers in healthcare facilities can make accessing care stressful and challenging for individuals with disabilities. Although clinics, hospitals, and medical offices should be fully accessible, this is often not the case.

Lack of Accessible Equipment: Many healthcare facilities lack accessible equipment like adjustable examination tables, wheelchair-friendly scales, or other devices that can make medical exams more comfortable and accessible.

A person who uses a wheelchair may find it difficult to transfer onto a standard examination table for a physical exam. Facilities without adjustable tables may not provide the comprehensive care needed, resulting in substandard evaluations.

Transportation Issues: Reaching medical appointments can also pose a challenge. Public transportation systems may lack full accessibility, and arranging alternative transportation can be costly or inconvenient, leading to missed appointments and delays in care.

Example: An individual with a visual impairment might rely on public transport but may face accessibility barriers on certain routes. Access to subsidized or specialized transportation services could alleviate these challenges.

Healthcare Provider Training and Awareness: A lack of training in disability-specific care is another common barrier. Many healthcare providers are not adequately prepared to address the unique healthcare needs of persons with disabilities, especially as aging-related issues overlap with disability-related needs.

Lack of Disability Sensitivity: Some healthcare providers may lack understanding of disability complexities, leading to misdiagnoses or overlooking the psychological aspects of care. Sensitivity training for healthcare providers can reduce these issues by promoting a more informed and empathetic approach to treatment.

Example: A person with epilepsy might feel misunderstood if their provider attributes symptoms solely to aging rather than considering the specific interactions between epilepsy and aging. Disability sensitivity training can ensure that providers take a holistic view of the patient's unique situation.

Strategies for Improving Access and Care

To overcome these barriers, persons with disabilities, caregivers, and healthcare providers can adopt specific strategies to create a more supportive and effective healthcare experience. This includes advocating for better care, understanding available resources, and leveraging existing support systems.

Self-Advocacy and Informed Healthcare Decisions: Persons with disabilities and their caregivers can benefit from becoming informed advocates. This involves understanding their rights, knowing what services are available, and effectively communicating with healthcare providers.

Understanding Patient Rights: Knowledge of patient rights under laws like the Americans with Disabilities Act (ADA) or Rights of Persons with Disabilities Act 2016 (RPwD Act 2016) in India or similar legislation is crucial. These laws protect against discrimination and guarantee necessary accommodations in healthcare settings.

Building a Knowledge Base: Being informed about one's medical condition, treatment options, and the healthcare system itself enables individuals to make empowered healthcare decisions. Researching conditions, asking questions during appointments, and seeking second opinions when necessary are all valuable strategies.

Example: A person with Parkinson's disease may research specialized exercise programs or diet adjustments that can support their condition in addition to medication. Being informed allows them to bring new ideas to their healthcare provider for consideration.

Navigating Healthcare Systems and Programs: Government programs, non-profit organizations, and advocacy groups can help individuals navigate healthcare complexities, access medical care, and find financial support.

Disability-Specific Organizations: Many organizations provide resources for specific disabilities, such as the Spinal Cord Injury Association, the National Federation of the Blind, or mental health advocacy groups. These organizations often offer information on healthcare rights and connections to specialists.

Example: An individual with cerebral palsy might connect with a cerebral palsy support group to find local specialists or therapists with relevant experience, ensuring they receive tailored care.

Case Management and Social Workers: Hospitals and healthcare organizations often provide case management services or access to social workers, who can help individuals with disabilities manage healthcare tasks, from finding transportation to completing insurance paperwork.

Example: A social worker could assist a person with autism in finding a specialist familiar with autism spectrum disorder in adults, ensuring their unique needs are addressed.

Promoting Better Communication with Healthcare Providers: Strong communication between individuals and healthcare providers is key to effective care. Patients and caregivers should feel empowered to discuss concerns, ask questions, and ensure their physical and emotional needs are considered.

Being Clear About Needs and Expectations: Patients should clearly communicate their specific needs during appointments, whether related to accessibility, mental health, or treatment options.

Example: A person with a hearing impairment might request that providers speak face-to-face to facilitate lip-reading or request written summaries of their visit. Communicating these needs upfront helps providers offer more effective care.

Building a Partnership with Providers: Working collaboratively with healthcare providers can lead to better outcomes. Patients and caregivers should feel like active participants in their healthcare decisions, promoting mutual respect and understanding.

Training and Education for Healthcare Providers

Improving healthcare for persons with disabilities requires that providers receive adequate training on disability-specific needs, especially for individuals facing the overlapping challenges of aging and disability.

Disability Sensitivity Training: Providers should undergo disability sensitivity training to understand the challenges their patients face. Such training promotes effective communication, empathy, and the avoidance of biases.

Example: A doctor working with patients with chronic pain could benefit from training on how to address pain management comprehensively, considering both physical and psychological aspects.

Incorporating Disability Education in Medical Schools and Continuing Education: Medical schools and continuing education programs should include disability-related healthcare topics. This includes understanding how certain disabilities progress, recognizing emotional distress, and learning about advancements in assistive technology.

Specialist Care for Aging with Disabilities: As individuals with disabilities age, they may require more specialized care to address chronic pain, mobility issues, and other progressive conditions that become more challenging in mid-life.

Encouraging Open Dialogue Between Professionals and Patients

Navigating the healthcare system successfully requires open and honest dialogue between patients and healthcare providers. Patients and caregivers should feel empowered to voice concerns, while providers should be open to addressing both physical and emotional health.

Creating a Safe Space for Conversation: Healthcare providers should encourage open discussions about both mental and physical health. Addressing the emotional toll of a mid-life crisis is essential, particularly for persons with disabilities who may face unique struggles.

Example: A primary care provider could ask open-ended questions to encourage a person with muscular dystrophy to discuss emotional challenges as well as physical symptoms, creating a supportive and comprehensive care plan.

Ongoing Conversations About Care Plans: As individuals age, their healthcare needs evolve. Regular conversations with providers about treatment goals, emerging concerns, and care adjustments help ensure that care remains effective and relevant.

Revisiting Care Plans: Periodically revisiting care plans allows providers and patients to assess what's working, adjust strategies, and set new goals, especially during mid-life when physical and emotional needs may shift.

Chapter 11: Sexuality and Intimacy in Mid-Life for Persons with Disabilities

Understanding Sexuality in Mid-Life

Sexuality is a fundamental aspect of human identity and well-being, influencing emotional health, personal satisfaction, and quality of life. During mid-life, sexuality often takes on new significance, as individuals re-evaluate their needs, desires, and relationships. For persons with disabilities, navigating sexuality at this stage may involve unique challenges and opportunities, shaped by physical changes, societal expectations, and personal reflection.

"Living with cerebral palsy, I've always struggled with feeling confident in my own skin, especially when it comes to intimacy. Now, at 45, with everyone around me talking about marriage, children, and companionship, I find myself wondering if I'll ever experience that kind of connection. The physical limitations I have make me self-conscious, and even though I yearn for closeness, I worry about rejection or being seen as 'too fragile' or 'too different.' Recently, I joined an online group where people with disabilities discuss relationships and sexuality, and it's given

The Importance of Sexuality for Well-Being: Sexuality is closely tied to self-esteem, emotional fulfilment, and relational satisfaction. For persons with disabilities, expressing sexuality can affirm their identity and challenge stereotypes that often desexualize individuals with disabilities. Intimacy and sexual expression provide not only physical pleasure but also emotional closeness, which can alleviate feelings of loneliness and enhance resilience in facing mid-life challenges. Many studies indicate that healthy sexual expression correlates with lower rates of depression and anxiety, emphasizing the role of sexuality in mental health.

How Mid-Life Crises Affect Sexual Identity and Desires: Mid-life often prompts a re-evaluation of personal identity, including sexual identity. Individuals may question their attractiveness, sexual capabilities, and desires, particularly as societal pressures and physical changes create new challenges. This period can bring about a "sexual renaissance," as some seek to explore new aspects of intimacy, while others may struggle with diminished libido or self-confidence.

A person with a physical disability who felt self-conscious about intimacy in younger years may now feel a renewed desire to embrace their sexuality, seeking new expressions of intimacy with their partner. Conversely, another person may struggle with self-worth and attractiveness, especially if physical changes have led to pain or discomfort during intimacy.

Intersection of Disability, Aging, and Sexuality: The interaction between disability and aging introduces unique complexities into one's sexual life. Age-related changes, such as decreased libido, hormonal shifts, and physical limitations, can affect sexual functioning and desire. For individuals with disabilities, these changes may feel more pronounced, and overcoming societal misconceptions that view them as asexual or uninterested in intimacy can add to the challenge. However, with open communication, education, and support, individuals can explore a sexuality that is fulfilling, adaptive, and authentic to their mid-life experience.

Challenges Faced by Persons with Disabilities

Mid-life brings distinct challenges to sexuality and intimacy, which are often amplified for persons with disabilities. Physical, psychological, and social factors influence confidence, relationship dynamics, and access to resources, often requiring individuals to find creative ways to maintain satisfying intimate lives.

Physical Challenges: Pain, Mobility, and Functional Impairments: Physical limitations—such as chronic pain, restricted mobility, and functional impairments—can directly impact one's ability to engage in traditional sexual activities. For individuals with disabilities, these challenges may be more complex, requiring adaptations or alternative approaches to intimacy.

Example: Someone with arthritis or a spinal cord injury may find certain physical positions uncomfortable or unsustainable. By exploring alternative positions, sensory-focused intimacy, or non-penetrative activities, couples can find ways to connect without physical strain. For example, activities like massage, sensory play, or shared relaxation exercises can be fulfilling alternatives to traditional sexual practices.

Psychological Barriers: Body Image, Confidence, and Shame: Body image concerns, feelings of inadequacy, and internalized shame can be significant barriers to sexual fulfilment. Society's emphasis on physical perfection can lead to self-doubt, particularly for individuals who may already feel marginalized due to their disability.

Example: A person with a visible disability may feel anxious about how their body is perceived, impacting their willingness to initiate or engage in intimacy. Developing a sense of self-acceptance, possibly with the support of a therapist, and engaging in open conversations with a partner about insecurities can help individuals feel more comfortable and confident in expressing their sexuality.

Social and Cultural Stigmas Around Sexuality and Disability: Society often marginalizes the sexuality of persons with disabilities, assuming they are less interested in or capable of intimate relationships. Cultural attitudes that treat disability as a barrier to sexual expression can lead to feelings of invisibility or inadequacy. For persons with disabilities, breaking free from these stereotypes is essential for self-worth and relational fulfilment.

Example: In some cultural contexts, individuals with disabilities may be discouraged from dating, marrying, or discussing sexual health. Challenging these stereotypes, whether through advocacy, storytelling, or community support, can foster a broader understanding of disability and sexuality, helping individuals reclaim their right to intimacy.

Communication Gaps with Partners and Healthcare Providers: Open discussions about sexuality are key to healthy relationships and sexual health, yet these conversations can be uncomfortable or avoided altogether. Some healthcare providers may lack training in discussing sexuality with persons with disabilities, leading to missed opportunities for support and guidance. Partners may also struggle with how to discuss intimacy issues, leading to misunderstandings or unmet needs.

A person with a disability might feel embarrassed or uncomfortable discussing sexual concerns with their doctor, fearing judgment or dismissal. They may also find it difficult to communicate their needs and preferences with a partner, which can impact the quality of intimacy in their relationship.

Navigating Sexual Health

Maintaining sexual health in mid-life is crucial for overall well-being and includes both proactive health management and open communication with healthcare providers. For persons with disabilities, addressing sexual health may require overcoming unique challenges, yet it remains essential for quality of life.

Sexual Health Concerns in Mid-Life: Common sexual health concerns during mid-life include reduced libido, erectile dysfunction, vaginal dryness, and hormonal changes, which can affect sexual enjoyment and intimacy. These issues may be exacerbated by disabilities that limit physical mobility, energy, or comfort. Sexual health concerns should be addressed holistically, considering both physical and emotional needs.

Example: An individual experiencing both chronic pain and hormonal changes may find it difficult to engage in traditional sexual activities. Exploring options like lubricants, hormone therapy, or adaptive equipment can make intimacy more enjoyable and accessible.

Accessing Sexual Health Services and Open Communication with Providers: Individuals with disabilities may encounter barriers in accessing sexual health services, including physical inaccessibility, provider bias, or discomfort discussing intimate issues. Building trust and communication with healthcare providers is essential for receiving quality care.

Example: Seeking out providers trained in disability and sexual health can improve the quality of care. Additionally, advocating for accessible healthcare facilities and educating providers about the unique sexual health needs of persons with disabilities can lead to more supportive and informed care.

Rebuilding Intimacy and Connection

Rebuilding or maintaining intimacy during mid-life requires flexibility, open-mindedness, and effective communication. For persons with disabilities, exploring alternative forms of intimacy and redefining relationship dynamics can help maintain a fulfilling and connected relationship.

Adapting to Physical Changes and Exploring Alternative Intimacy: Physical changes in mid-life may prompt individuals and their partners to experiment with different forms of intimacy that prioritize comfort, connection, and mutual enjoyment. Sensual touch, massage, and non-penetrative activities can offer pathways to intimacy without physical strain.

For instance, couples might explore sensual activities, such as giving each other massages or engaging in mindful touch practices that create connection without focusing on traditional sexual acts. These forms of intimacy can deepen emotional closeness and satisfaction.

Communication Strategies for Sexual Fulfilment: Open and honest communication is vital for a fulfilling sexual relationship. Partners should feel comfortable discussing preferences, limitations, and needs to foster mutual understanding and satisfaction.

Example: Regular, non-judgmental conversations about intimacy can help partners address challenges, explore new ideas, and affirm their commitment to each other. Creating a safe space for dialogue allows both partners to express themselves openly, enhancing trust and intimacy.

Counselling and Therapy for Sexual and Relationship Issues: Therapy can be invaluable for addressing psychological barriers to intimacy and helping individuals and couples improve their communication and connection. Couples counselling, sex therapy, and individual therapy provide spaces for exploring feelings related to body image, self-worth, and relationship dynamics.

A couple experiencing challenges with intimacy might attend couples counseling to explore underlying issues and learn new strategies for building emotional and physical closeness. Individual therapy can also support self-esteem and body acceptance, helping individuals feel more comfortable in their intimate lives.

Role of Caregivers and Healthcare Professionals

Caregivers and healthcare professionals play a vital role in supporting the sexual health and intimacy needs of persons with disabilities. Through empathetic guidance, education, and resource provision, they can help individuals and couples address sexuality openly and positively.

Supporting Healthy Sexuality Without Judgment: Caregivers and healthcare providers can support healthy sexuality by respecting the privacy and autonomy of persons with disabilities and addressing sexuality without judgment. This includes offering resources, listening without assumptions, and maintaining a respectful approach to conversations about intimacy.

Example: A caregiver can create a supportive environment by respecting boundaries around privacy and acknowledging the individual's right to pursue intimate relationships. Providing a safe, non-intrusive space fosters trust and allows individuals to feel comfortable discussing their needs.

Providing Resources and Offering Guidance: Healthcare professionals should provide resources on adaptive equipment, communication strategies, and sexual health. Recommendations for adaptive tools, specialized counsellors, or sexual health clinics can make a positive difference, ensuring individuals have access to support that respects their unique needs.

A healthcare provider might recommend specialized counselling or adaptive devices to support a person with disabilities in exploring their sexuality. By approaching sexuality as a normal and essential part of well-being, professionals can foster a comprehensive approach to care that addresses physical and emotional health.

Chapter 12: Coping with a Midlife Crisis for People with Disabilities

Embracing Midlife as a Time of Transformation

Midlife can be a period of profound change and reflection, especially for people with disabilities who may face unique societal and personal challenges. While a midlife crisis is often characterized by feelings of self-doubt and restlessness, it can also serve as a powerful time for transformation and self-discovery. With adaptive strategies, people with disabilities can navigate this stage with resilience, shifting from a period of crisis to one of growth and renewed purpose.

Let us go through some coping strategies to address the physical, emotional, and social challenges that people with disabilities may encounter during midlife. Embracing these techniques can help individuals not only manage midlife stress but also find new meaning and direction, leading to a fulfilling and empowered life.

Focusing on Self-Acceptance and Self-Compassion

Self-acceptance is essential for coping with a midlife crisis, especially for individuals with disabilities who may have experienced a lifetime of societal scrutiny or self-doubt. Embracing self-compassion during this period can alleviate feelings of inadequacy and frustration, supporting a healthier and more resilient outlook.

1. **Acknowledge Your Achievements:** Reflect on personal accomplishments, big or small, to counter feelings of unfulfillment. For instance, individuals with cerebral palsy or spinal cord injuries can celebrate their achievements in building independence or finding adaptive ways to pursue hobbies, which showcase resilience and adaptability.

2. **Challenge Negative Self-Talk:** Reframe negative thoughts with self-compassion. When feelings of inadequacy surface, remind yourself of the strength you have shown in managing life with a disability. A person with multiple sclerosis, for example, might reframe thoughts about limitations by focusing on their

perseverance in adapting to new health challenges.

3. Embrace Authenticity: Focus on what genuinely brings you joy and satisfaction, rather than societal expectations. A person with a visual impairment might choose to spend more time on creative pursuits that bring them joy, like music or writing, rather than striving to meet arbitrary milestones.

4. Practice Self-Compassion Techniques: Activities like mindfulness meditation, journaling, or positive self-affirmations can cultivate a kinder relationship with oneself. Engaging in these practices during moments of self-doubt fosters emotional resilience and acceptance.

Building and Strengthening Support Networks

A strong support network is crucial during a midlife crisis, especially for individuals with disabilities who may face additional challenges in accessing resources. Supportive communities offer not only emotional comfort but also practical advice and shared experiences.

1. Engage with Disability Advocacy Groups: Many advocacy groups provide resources and a sense of community. For example, the National Federation of the Blind offers programs tailored to individuals with visual impairments, providing a space for connection and shared understanding.

2. Seek Peer Support: Peer support groups, either in-person or online, create spaces for sharing struggles and successes. People with spinal cord injuries, for instance, might join online forums or local groups that address issues specific to living with mobility impairments, fostering solidarity and encouragement.

3. Reach Out to Family and Friends: Communicate openly with trusted family members or friends about your experiences. By discussing your needs, you can build stronger, more understanding relationships. This open communication is especially beneficial for individuals with "invisible" disabilities, such as chronic pain conditions, where loved ones may not fully understand the challenges faced.

4. Consider Professional Support: Speaking with a therapist knowledgeable about disability-related challenges can provide valuable coping tools. A therapist experienced in disability issues can help individuals with progressive conditions like Parkinson's disease or multiple sclerosis navigate the psychological impact of midlife changes.

Setting Realistic and Adaptable Goals

Midlife often involves re-evaluating life goals. For people with disabilities, goal-setting during this period can be empowering if approached with a realistic, adaptable mindset.

1. Reflect on Personal Values and Priorities: Instead of focusing on traditional societal milestones, consider what genuinely matters to you. For example, a person with muscular dystrophy might prioritize relationships, creative expression, or advocacy work, finding fulfillment in values that align with their personal strengths.

2. Break Down Goals into Achievable Steps: Set realistic goals that align with your needs and capabilities. If improving

physical health is a priority, someone with arthritis might start with small, manageable changes, such as gentle stretching exercises or short, daily walks, which can build confidence and foster a sense of accomplishment.

3. **Celebrate Progress, Not Perfection:** Recognize each step forward, no matter how small. For instance, an individual with chronic pain might celebrate a week of consistent self-care routines, reinforcing motivation and resilience.

4. **Be Open to Adjusting Goals:** Life circumstances and health may change, so being flexible with goals allows graceful adaptation. Remember that goals should evolve with you, serving as a guide rather than a strict measure of success.

Taking Care of Physical and Mental Health

Health is fundamental to coping with a midlife crisis, particularly for people with disabilities who may face added health considerations.

1. **Prioritize Physical Well-being:** Develop a routine that supports your physical health.

A person with a mobility impairment might focus on upper body exercises or adaptive yoga, which can be done at home to maintain strength and flexibility. Regular medical check-ups also ensure that emerging health concerns are addressed promptly.

2. **Address Mental Health Needs:** Midlife can be emotionally intense, making mental health support essential. Techniques such as cognitive-behavioural therapy (CBT) or mindfulness-based stress reduction can help manage symptoms of anxiety or depression. These approaches can be particularly useful for individuals with conditions like fibromyalgia, where mental health is closely linked to physical well-being.

3. **Manage Stress with Relaxation Techniques:** Practices like deep breathing, progressive muscle relaxation, or visualization exercises can help reduce stress and improve overall well-being. For individuals with autism spectrum disorder, these techniques can provide relief from sensory overloads often triggered by stress.

4. **Practice Good Sleep Hygiene:** Quality sleep is essential for managing stress and maintaining health. Individuals with disabilities may need tailored sleep solutions, such as specialized mattresses or sleep positions that minimize discomfort. A consistent bedtime routine and a relaxing environment can support better sleep quality.

Embracing Lifelong Learning and Personal Growth

One of the most empowering ways to cope with a midlife crisis is to pursue lifelong learning and new interests. This approach fosters curiosity, engagement, and self-discovery, which can reinvigorate one's sense of purpose.

1. **Explore New Hobbies or Interests:** Midlife is an ideal time to try new hobbies or revisit old passions. A person with a visual impairment might explore music, creative writing, or tactile arts like pottery, finding joy and fulfillment through expressive outlets.

2. **Seek Educational Opportunities:** Online courses and community programs make

learning accessible. For instance, someone with hearing impairments might benefit from online classes with closed captions, allowing them to learn new skills in a format that suits their needs.

3. **Focus on Personal Development:** Invest time in self-growth, whether through reading, creative pursuits, or participating in supportive communities. A person with PTSD, for example, might find solace and purpose in mindfulness practices or supportive networks focused on personal development.

4. **Volunteer or Mentor Others:** Sharing experiences and supporting others can bring a sense of fulfillment and connection. Volunteering or mentoring, especially within disability communities, can offer purpose and remind individuals of their strengths.

Practicing Gratitude and Mindfulness

Gratitude and mindfulness are transformative tools that can help manage the emotional challenges of a midlife crisis, fostering positivity and increased self-awareness.

151

1. Start a Gratitude Practice: Take time each day to reflect on things you're grateful for, even small moments of joy. For individuals dealing with chronic health issues, this practice can shift focus from what's challenging to what brings meaning.

2. Mindful Reflection: Engaging in mindfulness practices, such as meditation or mindful breathing, can improve emotional regulation and resilience, helping individuals approach midlife changes with greater clarity and acceptance.

3. Focus on the Present Moment: Mindfulness encourages individuals to stay present rather than dwell on past regrets or future worries. A person with PTSD might benefit from grounding exercises that focus on the present, providing a sense of calm and stability.

4. Engage in Positive Affirmations: Incorporate positive affirmations into daily routines to build self-compassion and counter feelings of self-doubt. For example, a person managing a progressive disability could use

affirmations to remind themselves of their strength and worth.

Chapter 13: Moving Forward with Resilience and Purpose

Navigating a midlife crisis is a deeply personal journey, especially for people with disabilities, and requires resilience, adaptability, and a supportive network. This chapter outlines practical strategies, from fostering self-acceptance and engaging with community resources to prioritizing health and embracing lifelong learning. Approaching midlife as a period of transformation allows individuals to find purpose, discover new strengths, and envision fresh possibilities for the future. Remember, midlife can be a time to evolve and thrive.

Reflecting on the Journey

Navigating mid-life is challenging for anyone, but for persons with disabilities, the physical, emotional, and social dimensions of this phase can present unique complexities. This book has delved into these challenges, offering practical strategies and solutions to empower individuals, caregivers, healthcare providers, and society to provide meaningful support.

While mid-life is often viewed as a period of decline, it can also be a time of growth, reinvention, and renewed purpose. By addressing the physical, emotional, and practical aspects of the mid-life experience, persons with disabilities can embrace change, discover new opportunities, and continue to live fulfilling, meaningful lives. In the Indian context, where community and family bonds are strong, mid-life can also be an opportunity to deepen these relationships and seek mutual support.

Personal Growth and Adaptation: Mid-life is an ideal time to re-evaluate personal goals, relationships, and career aspirations. For persons with disabilities, this phase may involve adapting to new physical or emotional realities, but it also offers opportunities for personal growth. Whether it's discovering new passions, engaging in creative pursuits, or redefining success on one's own terms, mid-life can be a period of reimagining the future.

Example: A person with visual impairment may find new ways to engage with the community through storytelling, advocacy, or public speaking, using their experiences to inspire others and raise awareness about disability rights.

Strengthening Relationships: Relationships with family, friends, and romantic partners can be tested during mid-life. However, they also have the potential to grow stronger. For many Indians, family support systems are integral, providing both practical assistance and emotional resilience. Open communication, role adaptation, and mutual respect can foster stronger, more supportive relationships.

Example: A person with a neurological condition like Parkinson's disease may find that their relationship with their spouse deepens as they navigate physical and emotional changes together, developing a shared resilience and understanding.

Building Resilience: Resilience has been a core theme throughout this book. Persons with disabilities and their caregivers often face adversity and have learned to adapt, a skill that becomes invaluable during mid-life. Strategies like seeking therapy, building a support network, and advocating for one's healthcare needs can help individuals thrive, even in the face of new challenges.

Looking Forward: Encouraging a Future of Growth and Well-Being

As persons with disabilities, caregivers, and healthcare professionals move forward from mid-life, it is important to envision a future focused on growth, connection, and well-being. While mid-life can be challenging, it is also a time for redefining personal goals, fostering meaningful relationships, and building a fulfilling life.

Embracing Change: Mid-life is a time of transition, and embracing these changes can lead to new experiences and self-discovery. By approaching this phase with adaptability and resilience, individuals can transform mid-life into an opportunity for growth and reinvention.

Strengthening Support Systems: Progress in mid-life requires a collaborative effort between individuals, families, caregivers, healthcare professionals, and society. Strong support systems foster resilience and confidence, ensuring that individuals with disabilities have the resources they need to thrive.

Empowerment and Advocacy: Empowerment is a crucial theme in navigating mid-life. Persons with disabilities should be empowered to advocate for their needs, whether in healthcare, the workplace, or personal relationships. This empowerment extends to society, which must continue to advocate for a more inclusive India that recognizes and values the contributions of persons with disabilities.

Final Reflection: A Journey of Transformation

It is essential to remember that mid-life is not just a period of challenges but also one of transformation. For persons with disabilities, navigating mid-life with resilience, adaptability, and support can lead to a fulfilling journey of self-discovery and growth. Indian society has a responsibility to continue evolving—ensuring equal opportunities, accessibility, and dignity for everyone. Moving forward with purpose, individuals with disabilities can continue to shape their lives, communities, and society, embracing mid-life as a stage of possibilities and new beginnings.

Key Takeaways

Each chapter of this book has provided insights into different aspects of the mid-life journey for persons with disabilities. Below are some key takeaways that can guide individuals, families, and support networks as they move forward.

- Understanding the Mid-Life Crisis: Mid-life crises can manifest uniquely for persons with disabilities, affecting physical health, mental well-being, and social relationships. Recognizing these challenges and taking proactive steps to manage them—whether through counseling, medical support, or social connections—can transform this period into an opportunity for growth and resilience.

- Supporting Caregivers: Caregivers are essential in the mid-life journey of persons with disabilities. However, they, too, need support. Caregiver burnout is a real concern, and it is crucial for caregivers to prioritize their own well-being, seek respite when needed, and balance caregiving with self-care.

- Navigating Healthcare: Access to healthcare is crucial for managing the physical and emotional challenges of mid-life. Regular check-ups, preventive care, and clear communication with healthcare providers help individuals stay on top of health concerns. Advocacy within the healthcare system can ensure that persons with disabilities receive comprehensive, respectful care, especially in India, where accessible healthcare is still evolving.

- Managing Disability-Specific Health Concerns: Different disabilities carry specific health risks as individuals age, such as musculoskeletal issues for those with mobility impairments or cognitive decline in people with neurological conditions. Regular screenings and proactive health management are essential for managing these conditions effectively.

- Financial and Career Planning: Financial security and career satisfaction are central concerns during mid-life. Persons with disabilities may face added challenges in sustaining employment, saving for the future, and managing healthcare costs. Planning for these financial realities early and exploring resources for financial support, such as government schemes or disability benefits, can alleviate stress.

- Societal Responsibility: Society plays a significant role in supporting persons with disabilities through mid-life. From ensuring inclusivity in public spaces to implementing policies that guarantee access to healthcare, education, and employment, society has a responsibility to create a supportive, inclusive environment that respects the rights and contributions of people with disabilities.

Resources and Further Support in the Indian Context

Accessing appropriate resources and support networks is vital for managing the challenges of mid-life. Below are recommended resources in the Indian context for individuals, caregivers, and healthcare providers.

- Disability Advocacy Organizations:
    - National Centre for Promotion of Employment for Disabled People (NCPEDP): Provides resources, advocacy, and support for the employment and empowerment of persons with disabilities.
    - The Spinal Foundation: Offers peer support, rehabilitation guidance, and resources for individuals with spinal cord injuries.
    - All India Federation of the Deaf (AIFD): Supports the deaf and hard-of-hearing community through resources, education, and advocacy.

- National Association for the Blind (NAB): Provides services and support for visually impaired individuals, including vocational training, rehabilitation, and advocacy.

- Caregiver Support Networks:

  - Caregiver Saathi: A support network offering resources, counseling, and guidance for caregivers of persons with disabilities and chronic illnesses.

  - Family Caregiving India: Provides information, support, and resources for family caregivers, helping them manage their caregiving responsibilities while prioritizing their own well-being.

- Healthcare Resources:

  - Ayushman Bharat - Pradhan Mantri Jan Arogya Yojana (PM-JAY): A government initiative providing health insurance coverage to economically disadvantaged families, including persons with disabilities, for essential medical services.

- o Rehabilitation Council of India (RCI): A statutory body that regulates training programs and maintains a registry of qualified rehabilitation professionals across India.

- o Swasth India: An organization focused on creating affordable and accessible healthcare services, providing resources for preventive care and treatment across India.

- Mental Health Support:

- o KIRAN Helpline (1800-599-0019): A national mental health helpline supported by the Ministry of Social Justice and Empowerment, offering counseling and support for mental health concerns.

- o Mind Matters Foundation: A mental health organization providing resources, counseling, and educational programs on mental well-being, including support for individuals with disabilities.

- Financial and Career Planning:

    - National Handicapped Finance and Development Corporation (NHFDC): Provides loans at concessional interest rates to persons with disabilities for self-employment ventures.

    - Skills Development Initiative Scheme: A program focused on vocational training to enhance employability for persons with disabilities, enabling them to achieve financial independence and career growth.

Appendix 1: Checklist for Regular Medical Screenings and Preventive Care for Persons with Disabilities

1. Physical Health Assessments

- Annual Physical Examination
    - General health check-up, including a review of existing conditions.
    - Ensure medication management and potential side effects are discussed.
- Blood Pressure Screening (at least annually, or more frequently if high blood pressure is an issue).
- Cholesterol and Blood Glucose Testing (every 1-3 years based on risk factors).
- Bone Density Test
    - Recommended for both men and women, especially with a history of limited mobility or wheelchair use, which can increase the risk of osteoporosis.

2. Cardiovascular Health

- EKG/Heart Health Screening (frequency depending on personal and family history).

- Lifestyle Counselling

  o Diet and physical activity assessment to reduce cardiovascular risks, even for those with mobility limitations.

3. Diabetes Screening

- Regular Blood Glucose Testing (annual or bi-annual for those with risk factors or family history).

- HbA1c Test to measure long-term blood sugar levels.

4. Cancer Screenings

- Breast Cancer Screening (Mammograms)

  o Women aged 40+ should consider regular screenings, with timing based on personal risk factors.

- Prostate Cancer Screening (for men over 50 or younger with risk factors).

- Colorectal Cancer Screening (starting at age 45 or earlier for those with family history).

- Skin Cancer Check (especially for those with limited mobility or sensation, which may delay noticing changes in the skin).

5. Musculoskeletal Health

- Physical Therapy or Mobility Assessments
    - Regular assessments by a physical therapist can help identify changes in mobility and prevent falls or injuries.

- Joint Health Checkups
    - People with certain disabilities are more susceptible to joint issues, such as arthritis, due to unusual strain on specific areas of the body.

6. Mental Health and Cognitive Screenings

- Depression and Anxiety Screening (annual or as needed).

- Cognitive Assessments if there are concerns about memory or cognitive decline.

- Support Services and Counseling for midlife transitions, stress management, and coping with disability-related challenges.

7. Sensory Health

- Hearing Tests (every 2-3 years or as needed).

- Vision Tests (annually or bi-annually), especially for individuals with conditions that may impact vision, such as diabetes.

8. Oral Health

- Dental Checkups and Cleanings (every 6 months).

- Oral Cancer Screening (for tobacco users or others at high risk).

9. Vaccinations and Immunizations

- Flu Vaccine (annually).

- COVID-19 Vaccinations and boosters as recommended.

- Pneumonia Vaccine (recommended for individuals over 50 or those with chronic conditions).

- Shingles Vaccine (recommended for adults over 50).

10. Pain and Sleep Management

- Pain Assessment

- Regular pain assessments, as individuals with disabilities may have chronic pain that impacts quality of life.

- Sleep Quality Assessment

    - Evaluate sleep patterns and address sleep disorders, as poor sleep can worsen midlife symptoms.

11. Social and Lifestyle Support

- Social Engagement Check-in

    - Address potential social isolation, which can impact mental health.

- Assistive Device Check (for those using wheelchairs, walkers, or other aids)

    - Ensure devices are functioning properly and meet current needs.

- Community Resources and Support Groups

    - Connect individuals with disability support networks to address midlife challenges and transitions.

Appendix 2: Additional Tips for Preventive Care

- Encourage a Healthy Diet tailored to specific needs, especially if mobility is limited.

- Exercise Program – adapted physical activity is essential for cardiovascular and musculoskeletal health.

- Regular Monitoring of Medication Side Effects as new symptoms may arise with age or changing health conditions.

- Develop a Personalized Health Plan with healthcare providers to address individual risk factors.

Tips for Preventing Caregiver Burnout During Midlife Crisis of Disabled Loved Ones

1. Acknowledge Your Feelings and Limits

   - Accept that caregiving can be emotionally taxing, especially when witnessing a loved one experience a midlife crisis.

- o Recognize that it's normal to feel overwhelmed, frustrated, or even resentful at times. These emotions do not diminish your dedication.

2. **Set Realistic Expectations**

- o Avoid setting overly ambitious goals or expecting perfection from yourself. Small, achievable tasks are often more manageable and effective.

- o Communicate openly with your loved one about what you can and cannot do. Clear boundaries can prevent misunderstandings and resentment.

3. **Seek Support from Family and Friends**

- o Don't be afraid to ask for help or delegate tasks to other family members or friends. This can include help with household chores, errands, or respite care.

- o Encourage your loved one to participate in community programs, day centers, or disability support groups where they can socialize and engage in activities.

4. **Utilize Professional Resources**

   o Consider working with a therapist or counselor to process your emotions and manage stress.

   o Explore options for professional caregiving support or respite care to give yourself regular breaks.

5. **Join a Caregiver Support Group**

   o Connecting with other caregivers can be immensely validating and comforting. Support groups offer practical advice, emotional support, and a safe space to share experiences.

   o Some groups focus specifically on caregivers for people with disabilities, which can help address unique challenges.

6. **Practice Self-Compassion**

   o Remind yourself that caring for someone else is a big responsibility, and it's okay to feel a range of emotions.

    ○ Celebrate small victories and allow yourself to feel proud of the care you provide.

Suggestions for Creating a Self-Care Routine for Caregivers

Creating a self-care routine can help you recharge and stay balanced. Here's a step-by-step guide to building a sustainable routine:

1. Start with the Basics: Physical Health

- Sleep Hygiene: Aim for 7-8 hours of sleep. Try to go to bed and wake up at the same time daily, creating a wind-down routine to help signal bedtime.

- Balanced Diet: Eating regular, balanced meals fuels your body. Keep healthy snacks on hand for quick energy when time is limited.

- Regular Exercise: Aim for at least 20-30 minutes of physical activity most days, even if it's just a walk. Exercise can reduce stress and improve energy levels.

2. Schedule "Me Time" Every Day

- Set aside at least 15-30 minutes daily for something you enjoy. This could be reading, meditating, gardening, or even watching a favourite show.

- Treat this time as non-negotiable. Remind yourself that you deserve a break just as much as anyone else.

3. Incorporate Mindfulness and Relaxation Techniques

- Mindful Breathing: Spend a few minutes each day focusing on your breath. This can be as simple as taking a few deep breaths or using a breathing app to guide you.

- Meditation or Yoga: Practices like yoga or meditation can help you center yourself and reduce anxiety. Apps like Calm or Headspace offer guided meditations for busy caregivers.

- Gratitude Practice: Before bed, write down three things you're grateful for, even on difficult days. This can help shift your focus to the positive.

4. Stay Connected Socially

- Make time for social interactions, even if it's a quick phone call with a friend or family member. Caregiving can be isolating, so connecting with others can help you feel supported.

- Schedule regular social activities outside of caregiving when possible—such as coffee with a friend or a book club meeting.

5. Practice Creative Outlets and Hobbies

- Engage in a creative activity that brings you joy, such as painting, writing, cooking, or crafting. Creative expression can be a powerful way to release stress.

- Even if it's only once a week, prioritizing this activity can provide a mental escape from caregiving responsibilities.

6. Set and Enforce Boundaries

- Schedule time away from caregiving duties to prevent emotional and physical exhaustion. Whether it's a weekend getaway or a simple afternoon off, make it a regular practice.

- Communicate boundaries clearly with family members and your loved one, if possible, to ensure everyone understands and respects your time.

7. Keep a Journal to Process Emotions

- Journaling can be therapeutic, helping you to process difficult emotions without judgment. Consider writing about your day, feelings, or even small moments of joy.

- Use a journal to track progress in your self-care routine, as it can help you see improvements over time and adjust as needed.

8. Celebrate Small Wins

- Take time to acknowledge even small achievements or positive moments in your caregiving role.

- Reward yourself with something special occasionally, whether it's a favorite treat, a new book, or a relaxing bath.

9. Focus on What You Can Control

- Caregiving can be unpredictable, and many aspects are outside your control. Focus on what you can manage, like your reactions, self-care, and outlook.

- Recognize that setbacks happen, and don't be too hard on yourself when things don't go as planned.

10. Use Respite Care Regularly

- Regularly schedule time off from caregiving by utilizing respite care options if available. Respite care offers temporary relief, allowing you to take a break to recharge.

- Look for community organizations or professional services that provide short-term caregiving support.

Sample Self-Care Routine for Caregivers

- Morning: 10 minutes of stretching or yoga, followed by a nutritious breakfast.

- Midday: Take a 15-minute walk outside or do a quick mindfulness practice to recharge.

- Afternoon: Enjoy a healthy snack, and schedule a few minutes to call a friend or family member.

- Evening: Write in a gratitude journal, read a few pages of a book, or do a relaxing activity like knitting or listening to music.

- **Before Bed:** Reflect on your day with a few minutes of deep breathing or meditation to wind down.

Appendix 3: For Healthcare Professionals: Comprehensive Care for Midlife Persons with Disabilities

1. Guidelines for Creating Comprehensive Care Plans for Persons with Disabilities in Midlife

When developing a care plan for individuals with disabilities entering midlife, healthcare professionals should consider the complex intersection of physical, mental, and social health. Here are some essential guidelines to create an effective, individualized care plan:

A. Conduct a Thorough Assessment

- Medical History Review: Evaluate the individual's full medical history, focusing on existing disabilities, any chronic conditions, and potential age-related health risks.

- Functional Assessment: Assess physical, sensory, and cognitive abilities, noting any changes in functionality that could impact daily living and independence.

- Mental Health Evaluation: Screen for mental health issues like anxiety, depression, and stress, which may intensify in midlife due to physical limitations, social changes, or personal losses.

- Social and Environmental Factors: Examine the social support network, living environment, and accessibility needs. Consider any family dynamics, potential caregiver burnout, and community resources available.

B. Set Realistic and Personalized Health Goals

- Collaborative Goal Setting: Work with the individual and their family or caregivers to establish achievable health and lifestyle goals that align with their abilities and needs.

- Quality of Life Focus: Emphasize goals that improve daily life quality, such as pain management, mobility maintenance, and mental well-being.

- Self-Management: Encourage independence and self-management for achievable health tasks, fostering a sense of control and autonomy where possible.

C. Design Individualized Care Interventions

- Physical Health Interventions:

  - Pain Management: Create a pain management plan, which may include physical therapy, medication, or alternative therapies like acupuncture or relaxation techniques.

  - Exercise and Mobility: Develop an adapted exercise program tailored to their physical abilities, focusing on improving mobility, cardiovascular health, and muscle strength.

  - Preventive Screenings: Schedule regular screenings for common midlife health risks (e.g., cardiovascular health, cancer screenings, diabetes).

- Mental Health Support:

  - Counseling and Therapy: Incorporate mental health support into the care plan, such as regular counseling or therapy sessions, to address issues like depression, anxiety, and feelings of isolation.

- o Social Connection: Encourage involvement in social or community activities that are accessible and provide a sense of belonging.

- Lifestyle and Environmental Adjustments:

  - o Assistive Technology: Consider tools and technology that support independence, such as mobility aids, adaptive devices, or home modifications.

  - o Healthy Lifestyle Habits: Provide guidance on nutrition, sleep hygiene, and stress management techniques that are feasible within their limitations.

D. Coordinate a Multidisciplinary Team Approach

- Collaborative Care: Involve specialists as needed, including physical and occupational therapists, mental health professionals, social workers, and primary care providers.

- Caregiver Involvement: Include caregivers in care planning discussions to ensure they feel supported and have the resources they need.

- Regular Follow-Ups: Schedule periodic evaluations to review progress and adjust the care plan based on the individual's changing needs or new challenges.

E. Encourage Autonomy and Empowerment

- Respect the individual's preferences and goals, allowing them to make choices regarding their care to the greatest extent possible.

- Provide educational resources and training for self-care practices, encouraging the person with a disability to be an active participant in their health journey.

2. Screening Tools for Mental Health Concerns in Persons with Disabilities

Individuals with disabilities can experience mental health concerns that may be amplified during midlife. Using appropriate screening tools tailored to their specific needs is crucial for accurate assessment. Here are some recommended tools:

A. General Mental Health Screening Tools

- PHQ-9 (Patient Health Questionnaire-9):
    - Purpose: Screens for depression severity.
    - Adaptation for Disabilities: The PHQ-9 can be administered in different formats (self-reported, verbally by a provider) and is effective for adults with mild cognitive impairments.
- GAD-7 (Generalized Anxiety Disorder-7):
    - Purpose: Measures the severity of anxiety.
    - Use in Disabilities: Works well for identifying anxiety symptoms in individuals who can understand and respond to the questions directly.

B. Cognitive Function and Neuropsychological Screening

- Mini-Mental State Examination (MMSE):

- Purpose: Assesses cognitive impairment.
    - Adaptation: Though originally designed for general populations, it may need adjustments for persons with sensory disabilities.
- Montreal Cognitive Assessment (MoCA):
    - Purpose: Screens for mild cognitive impairment and dementia.
    - Use for Disabilities: The MoCA is suitable for individuals with physical disabilities and includes versions that account for visual impairment.

C. Disability-Specific Screening Tools

- Beck Depression Inventory-II (BDI-II):
    - Purpose: Assesses symptoms of depression.
    - Use for Physical Disabilities: This tool can help capture physical manifestations of depression, like fatigue, often mistaken for symptoms related to physical disabilities.

- Adaptive Behavior Assessment System (ABAS-3):

    o Purpose: Evaluates adaptive behavior and independent living skills.

    o Use for Developmental Disabilities: Helps assess how mental health impacts adaptive functioning, especially useful for adults with intellectual or developmental disabilities.

D. Specialized Tools for Assessing Psychosocial Aspects

- Quality of Life in Neurological Disorders (Neuro-QOL):

    o Purpose: Measures health-related quality of life in individuals with neurological disorders, covering domains like depression, anxiety, and social relationships.

    o Use: Suitable for people with multiple sclerosis, spinal cord injury, and other disabilities affecting quality of life in midlife.

- Life Satisfaction Questionnaire (LiSat-11):

- Purpose: Assesses satisfaction across multiple life areas, such as health, employment, and family.

  - Use for Physical Disabilities: This tool is useful for understanding life satisfaction and identifying areas where mental health support may be needed.

E. Social Isolation and Support Assessment

- Lubben Social Network Scale (LSNS):

  - Purpose: Evaluates social support and identifies individuals at risk of social isolation.

  - Use in Midlife: Effective for midlife individuals who may experience social isolation due to mobility restrictions or sensory impairments.

- Duke Social Support Index (DSSI):

  - Purpose: Measures the amount and type of social support.

  - Use for Disabilities: Helps identify the degree of support available, especially for those who rely heavily on caregivers or family.

Guidance for Implementation

- Choose Accessible Formats: When administering screening tools, consider alternative formats, such as verbal interviews or digital adaptations, to accommodate sensory and physical limitations.

- Provide Trauma-Informed Care: Many individuals with disabilities have experienced trauma or discrimination. Be sensitive to their background and adapt the approach to avoid causing distress.

- Regularly Reevaluate: Mental health needs can fluctuate, so consider regular screenings, especially during midlife, when personal identity, self-worth, and lifestyle can shift significantly.

Appendix 4: Further Reading and Research

1. Disability and Aging Books

"Aging with Disability: A Guide for Healthcare Professionals" by Bryan J. Kemp and Laura Mosqueda

This book offers an in-depth look at the intersection of aging and disability, providing healthcare professionals with strategies for addressing the unique needs of aging individuals with disabilities.

"Disability and Aging: Learning from Both to Empower the Lives of Older Adults" by Andrew Achenbaum and others

A multidisciplinary examination of how disability affects the aging process, this book focuses on enhancing the quality of life through research and best practices.

"The Disability Bioethics Reader" by Joel Michael Reynolds and Christine Wieseler

While not solely focused on aging, this reader provides insights into the ethical and social considerations of disability over the lifespan, which is useful for understanding aging with a disability.

Research Papers

"Aging with physical disability in Canada: Personal perspectives on health and aging" by M.J. Zwicker and H. Emery (2017)

This study provides first-hand accounts from Canadians aging with disabilities, exploring how disability impacts physical and mental health in later life.

"Ageing and disability: The paradoxical effects of ageing on functional status among older disabled adults" by H.L. Wong and C.Y. Leung (2019)

This paper examines the relationship between aging and disability, highlighting how physical limitations may change with age and impacting quality of life.

Articles

"Aging with Disability: Implications for Individuals and Health Care Providers" by Edward J. Roy and colleagues in the American Journal of Physical Medicine & Rehabilitation (2020)

An article that discusses the medical, psychological, and social challenges of aging with a disability and offers guidance for healthcare providers.

"Aging and Disability: Beyond Stereotypes to Inclusion" by the World Health Organization (WHO)

This article from the WHO explores the myths surrounding aging and disability, focusing on the need for inclusion and improved quality of life.

2. Midlife Psychological and Physical Health Books

"Midlife: A Philosophical Guide" by Kieran Setiya

Setiya's book provides a philosophical perspective on navigating midlife challenges, including identity, meaning, and self-acceptance. It addresses both the psychological and physical aspects of midlife.

"The Middle Passage: From Misery to Meaning in Midlife" by James Hollis

A Jungian approach to understanding the midlife transition, this book discusses the emotional and psychological aspects of midlife, which are relevant for those with disabilities and their caregivers.

"How to Age" by Anne Karpf

A comprehensive look at how to approach aging with resilience and positivity. This book discusses psychological and physical health, relevant for midlife individuals with or without disabilities.

Research Papers

"Mental Health and Well-being of Persons with Disabilities in Midlife" by S. O. Hampton and K. M. Prendergast (2018)

This study explores the mental health challenges unique to people with disabilities during midlife, with recommendations for mental health professionals.

"Aging, disability, and midlife physical health: A framework for assessment and intervention" by B. Zablotsky and R. Erickson (2019)

This paper proposes a framework for assessing physical health needs in midlife, particularly focusing on individuals with lifelong disabilities.

Articles

"Midlife Health Crisis: Physical and Psychological Challenges for the Disabled Population" by J. T. Ward in Health Psychology Review (2021)

An article that examines the unique challenges faced by individuals with disabilities in midlife,

193

covering both psychological and physical health issues.

"Midlife and Disability: Navigating a Complex Health Landscape" by National Institute on Aging (NIA)

This article by the NIA provides a broad overview of the midlife challenges for people with disabilities, focusing on both health maintenance and quality of life.

3. Caregiving Strategies Books

"The Caregiving Trap: Solutions for Life's Unexpected Changes" by Pamela D. Wilson

This book provides practical advice for caregivers, covering the emotional, physical, and logistical challenges they face, including a section on midlife caregiving.

"A Family Caregiver's Guide to Planning and Decision Making for the Elderly" by Harold G. Koenig and Andrew T. Care

Though primarily about elderly caregiving, this guide is helpful for midlife caregivers, especially those caring for loved ones with disabilities.

"The Conscious Caregiver: A Mindful Approach to Caring for Your Loved One Without Losing Yourself" by Linda Abbit

This book takes a mindful approach to caregiving, offering strategies to prevent burnout, maintain self-care, and manage stress.

Research Papers

"Supporting Caregivers of Persons with Disabilities: A Midlife Perspective" by A.L. Scharlach and B. Esterson (2018)

This research paper delves into the specific needs of caregivers for midlife adults with disabilities, including social support and coping strategies.

"The Role of Social Support in Preventing Burnout Among Midlife Caregivers" by L. Martinez and K. Patel (2020)

This paper discusses the importance of social support networks and explores strategies that caregivers can use to prevent burnout.

Articles

"Caregiver Burnout: Strategies for Coping with Midlife Challenges" by the Family Caregiver Alliance (FCA)

This article offers advice for managing the stress of caregiving during midlife, focusing on self-care and stress reduction techniques.

"Aging Parents and Midlife Caregivers: Reducing the Risk of Burnout" by the American Psychological Association (APA)

While focused on elder care, this article provides useful insights for caregivers in midlife, including boundary setting and mental health care.

About The Author

An author, trainer, professional counsellor, social worker, motivational speaker and disability rights advocate, Dr Abha Khetarpal, is a National Award winner, felicitated by the President of India and one of the 100 Women Achievers in India. She is the first woman from India to be honoured with Henry Viscardi Achievement Award. She writes extensively on disability issues and has developed various curricula for online courses on disability.